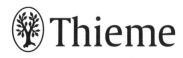

About the Authors

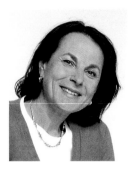

Françoise Wilhelmi de Toledo, MD, was born in Geneva and did her first fasting when she was 17. Since then, she has fasted every year out of conviction and passion. Being a physician, she is, together with her husband Raimund Wilhelmi, responsible for the medical concept of the Buchinger Fasting Clinics at Lake Constance, Germany and Marbella, Spain. The author is committed to the scientific documentation of fasting therapies. She regularly counsels fasting retreats for various institutions. The author has published numerous scientific papers on the subject of fasting. She has two sons.

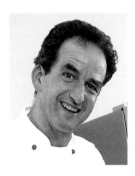

Hubert Hohler has been chef at the Buchinger Fasting Clinic at Lake Constance, Germany since 1997. One of his responsibilities is elaborating the building-up phase, that is, the return to a healthy nutrition. But he also conjures up delicious four-course menus containing only a few hundred calories. He is particularly passionate about organic wholefoods, high-quality and regional products, as well as the slow-food movement.

Dedication

I dedicate this book to my husband Raimund Wilhelmi, grandson of Dr. Otto Buchinger, to my mother-in-law Maria Buchinger-Wilhelmi, and our family, who have served therapeutic fasting for three generations.

Acknowledgement

I would like to thank the staff of the Buchinger Fasting Clinics at Lake Constance, Germany, and Marbella, Spain, for their therapeutic competence and dedication to the fasting patients from all over the world visiting Überlingen since 1953 and Marbella since 1973. I am so grateful to Marc Cziczek, Anne Bleick, Dr. Heinz Fahrner, Helmut Klepzig, Christianne Méroz, and Dr. Myriam Lejeune for their precious support.

About the Title

The Buchinger Amplius fasting method is the contemporary version of the fasting method that Dr. Otto Buchinger (1878–1966) developed and practiced as a means of healing himself of acute rheumatic fever.
His daughter, Maria Buchinger, his son-in-law, Helmut Wilhelmi, as well as the author and three generations of coworkers of the fasting clinics at Lake Constance, Germany, and Marbella, Spain and their medical followers, actualize and update the Buchinger Amplius Fasting Program for therapy, prevention, and as a basis for a safe spiritual exercise. The Latin word *amplius* means »Ahead! Forward!,« which was the motto of Otto Buchinger. The Buchinger Amplius fasting method is based on the *Guidelines for Therapeutic Fasting*, which the author wrote and published in 2002 together with other international experts.

Françoise Wilhelmi de Toledo, MD

Hubert Hohler

Therapeutic Fasting: The Buchinger Amplius® Method

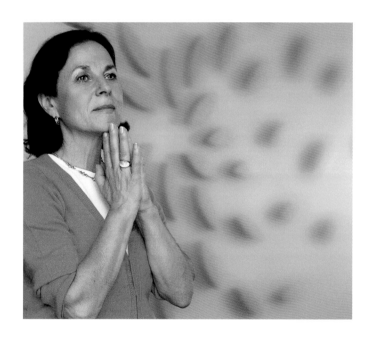

Thieme

Stuttgart · New York

Library of Congress Cataloging-in-Publication Data is available from the publisher.

This book is an authorized translation of the German edition published and copyrighted 2010 by TRIAS Verlag, Stuttgart. Title of the German edition: Buchinger Heilfasten. Die Original-Methode.

Translator: Ruth Gutberlet, Chom, NCTMB, Cochem, Germany.

Picture Credits
Corel Stock: p. 5 right; Chris Meier, Stuttgart: pp. 111, 113, 115, 117, 119, 121, 123, 125, 132, 135, 136, 138, 141, 143, 144, 146, 149, 150; Medioimages: pp. X, XII, 50, 104; Jens van Zoest, Wuppertal: pp. II, III, V–VIII, 3, 5 left, 6, 8, 9, 12, 13, 15, 16, 19, 21, 24, 27, 29, 31, 41, 42, 44, 45, 47, 49, 55–57, 60, 62, 64–70, 74, 75, 77–79, 81, 84, 86, 88–91, 93–97, 101–103, 106–109, 127, 129, 130, 153; Sabine Seifert: p. 32.

© 2012 Georg Thieme Verlag,
Rüdigerstrasse 14, 70469 Stuttgart, Germany
http://www.thieme.de
Thieme New York, 333 Seventh Avenue,
New York, NY 10001, USA
http://www.thieme.com

Cover design: Thieme Publishing Group
Typesetting by Cyclus Media Produktion, Stuttgart, Germany
Printed in Germany by AZ Druck und Datentechnik GmbH

ISBN 978-3-13-160361-6   4 5 6

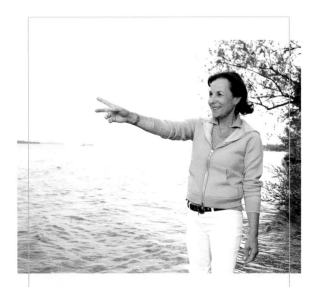

Letting Go of the Superfluous
Fasting is a natural ability, whereby the body automatically taps into its reserves. Trust and let go; the body will rid itself of superfluous lipids and metabolic waste:

Fasting from Conviction and Passion
Sharing very personal experiences, the author depicts fasting as a recurring theme in her life:

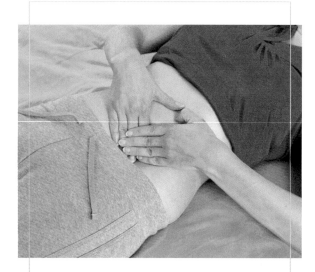

Thorough Detoxification

Not only will the gastrointestinal tract reshape during therapeutic fasting, but all cells of the body are detoxified. You can support elimination:

Breaking the Fast

Return to eating gently and consciously:

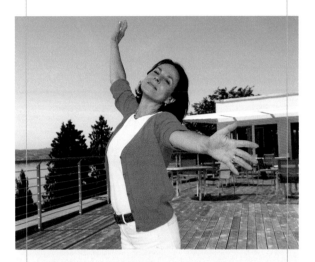

Lifting-Off—The Spiritual Dimension
Initially, many try fasting for physical reasons. But increasing fasting experience also brings about increasing awareness and presence. During the temporary abstention of food, mundane burdens dissolve and horizons broaden:

Feeling Well and Relaxing through Yoga
On pages 65–69, you will find some simple yoga exercises that are particularly helpful during fasting.

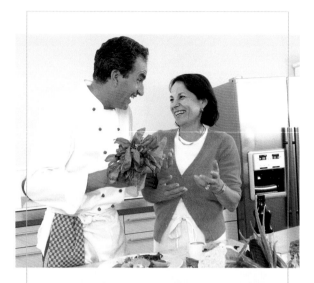

Pleasure from Eating is Top Priority

The dietary change following the fast is not about abstention; on the contrary, it is about richer and more intense experiences. On pages 106–109 and 126–129, the authors provide you with valuable suggestions for a healthy and diverse diet.

Preparing Delicious Low-calorie Food

The chef of the biggest European fasting center, on Lake Constance, will tell you how to successfully combine delicious food and healthy eating—his recipes are creative and rich in vital nutrients:

Service

Adresses

Buchinger Fasting Clinic
Lake Constance
Wilhelm-Beck-Str. 27
88662 Überlingen
Germany
Phone: +49 (0)7551-807-0
info@buchinger.com
www.buchinger.com

Clinica Buchinger Marbella
Avda. Buchinger s/n
29602 Marbella
Spain
Phone: +34 952-764300
clinica@buchinger.es
www.buchinger.es

Resources

Brantschen N. Fasting: What, Why, How. New York: The Crossraod Publising Company; 2010.

Guidelines for Therapeutic Fasting
www.maria-buchinger-foundation.com
www.amplius.com

Orbach S. On Eating. Change your Eating Change your Life. London: Penguin; 2002.

Servan-Schreiber D. Anticancer: A New Way of Life. New York: Penguin; 2008.

Tolle E. The Power of Now. A Guide to Spiritual Enlightenment. Hodder & Stoughton: London; 2001.

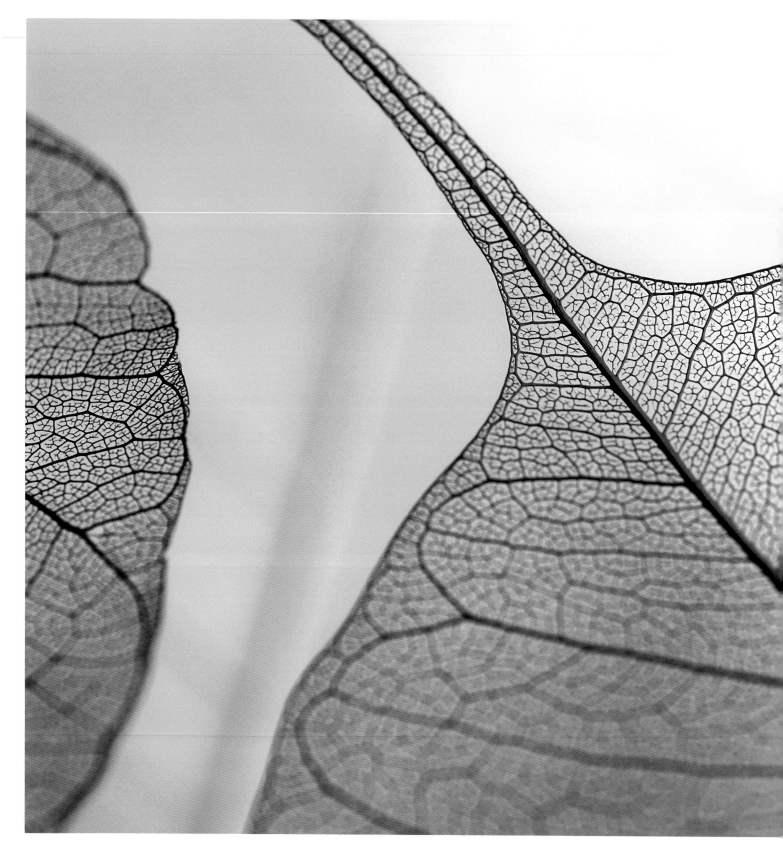

About this Book

This book invites you to rediscover your natural ability to fast. The fasting program sleeps in your genes and awakens when you voluntarily cease eating for a period of time and live off your fat reserves. You can do it! You will be surprised how simple it is if it is done the right way.

Fasting is an experience. It provides us with space and time. It leads to the development of awareness. It allows access to a deep and simple joy found within nature, communication, silence, and in being present. It cleanses body and soul and releases unimagined energies. Subsequently, eating can be truly relished again. The senses are awakened and more receptive. One's own existence is viewed from a new perspective.

But—how to do it the right way? Whether you fast in a clinic or at home, certain rules and rituals, which we convey in this book, must be observed. Fasting is an art. I would like to accompany you on this fascinating exploration so that, step by step, you regain your ability to fast, without apprehension but with reverence.

The Buchinger Amplius fasting method is the holistic method presented in this book. It is a contemporary and safe way of fasting, based on medical and physiological knowledge and extensive experience. This program is the further development of Dr. Otto Buchinger's (1878-1966) method by three generations of medical family members and co-workers. His daughter, Maria Buchinger, developed the human social dimension of this program and his son-in-law, Helmut Wilhelmi, gave the program the entrepreneurial push to achieve international renown. Their work has carried on and in 2002, a group of European medical fasting experts together with the author published the *Guidelines for Therapeutic Fasting* upon which this book is built. If you would like to rediscover the art of fasting and safely experience the gifts of voluntary abstention, please continue reading and let me be your guide.

Françoise Wilhelmi de Toledo, MD

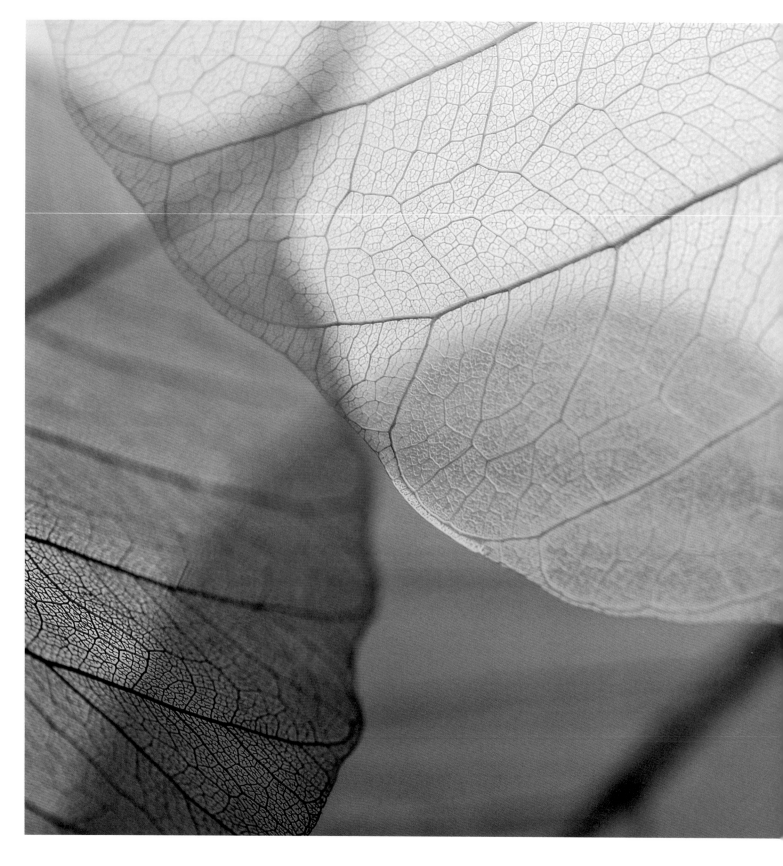

Fasting—The Basics

Fasting is a natural process. In times of food shortage, animals live off their fat reserves and humans can do the same. Not only is the voluntary temporary abstention from food intake a method to normalize body weight, it is also an opportunity for a metabolical reset, a cleansing of the body, and a way to get in touch with our spiritual dimension.

Fasting is Natural

Nature fasts, animals fast, and humans also have the ability to switch their metabolism to fat-reserve burning. As soon as food intake is discontinued, the body automatically switches from external to internal nutrition. Fasting is not something that we do, but it is something that we allow to happen. This book describes a fasting method, the Buchinger Amplius fasting program, which addresses the human being in all its dimensions.

Therapeutic fasting is a modified fast, including vegetable soups, freshly squeezed fruit and vegetable juices, herbal tea with a small amount of honey (approximately 250 kcal), as well as plenty of water. These supplements »boost« the fasting metabolism. They stimulate the burning of fat reserves and facilitate the sparing use of body proteins. At the same time, natural vitamins and minerals are supplied. The concept, as explained below, can turn a fasting period into an unforgettable experience.

The Concept of the Buchinger Amplius Fasting Method

- The concept of the Buchinger Amplius fasting method is based on medical knowledge but also includes the other two traditional dimensions of fasting: the spiritual and the social dimensions. When a person fasts, the body benefits; if it is a collective fast, the fasting community grows together. In either case, fasting eases the approach to spiritual experience.
- The journey into the »fasting space« is accomplished in four steps: planning, preparing, fasting, and building-up.
- Seven pillars uphold and unfold the healing power of fasting for body, soul, and spirit: balance between rest and movement, stimulation of elimination processes, adjuvant therapies, professional and compassionate care, individual treatments, and »food for the soul.«

In the fasting clinics at Lake Constance and Marbella, a professional team from different therapeutic areas—medicine, nutrition, psychology, physical therapy, physical exercise

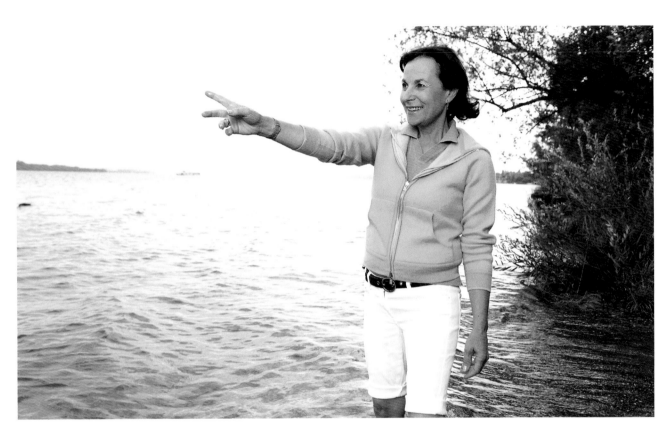

and body care, as well as health education, culture, and spirituality—attend to the fasting guests.

What are the rewards of temporary abstention from culinary pleasure? Cleansing, clearing out the body, mobilization of your healing power, general relief, as well as vitalization, energy build-up, renewed strength, and internal harmony. You treat your metabolism, your liver, and your digestive tract to a vacation!

Regular fasting, in terms of the voluntary and temporary abstention from food, can be an important tool for mental hygiene. Depressed mood can be prevented by retreating regularly and by consciously deliberating whether one's vision of life is lived, if the zest for life is still felt, if one brings out the best (in oneself), or if something needs to be adjusted. Ideally, all this can take place in harmony. Frequently, life crises or diseases force these adjustments. Deliberate

fasting possibly spares us such detours.

» Fasting or ›enduring the fast‹—when our being goes along, gaining deeper insights, understanding how to approach the fast …, saying ›yes‹ to it … allows us to be full of vigor when fasting.«
Niklaus Brantschen, Swiss Jesuit

Fasting is just as natural as sleeping, giving birth, breast-feeding, or dying.

A hectic lifestyle and excessive over-thinking may complicate and interfere with these natural functions. To gain knowledge about the process helps to reduce fear and allows these events to take their natural course, for example, as in prenatal classes for pregnant women.

I would like to explain what happens in the body when you temporarily and voluntarily abstain from food. This way, you can begin the »fasting program« (or »nutritional program II«) with trust and confidence. You will also be able to actively direct its course. You can be trusting because the body's stored fat supplies are to a fasting person what food is to an eating person. You are not going to be hungry, weak, or bored. As a matter of fact it will be the opposite.

same as starvation, therefore, we have decided to use the term fasting with regard to animals as well—notwithstanding that the concept of voluntariness cannot be taken literally here.

The Penguin, a Fasting Professional

At this point I would like to introduce to you the king penguin (*Aptenodytes patagonicus*). Since the 1970s, our good friend, Dr. Yvon Le Maho and his research team have employed the latest in technology to explore the penguin's life in the iciness of the Antarctic. The king penguin lives solely off fish and shellfish. It has to travel inland in order to breed, up to 180 km away from the ocean. Chubby, well-fed males and females migrate to their breeding grounds. For the next few weeks, they will live off their reserves: fat, micronutrients, and some protein, which they use up rather sparingly, just like humans do. King penguins search for their »loved one« while fasting and mate when they find them. Still fasting, the female lays an egg after 5 to 6 weeks. The adaptability of the protein structures of a fasting organism is vividly demonstrated by this ability to produce an egg weighing 400 g from the body's own reserves. Fasting king penguins are able to build up their summer feathers while molting, using only 1 kg of their body's own protein!

Nature Fasts

» The ability to fast is an evolutionary adaptation to the climatic conditions on our planet. In our temperate climate zone, we are privileged to live through the different seasons. Let us imagine life before the invention of refrigerators and food preservation technologies: the summer sun lets fruits, fresh vegetables, and many other foods grow. The colorful autumn is the time of fruit and grain harvest, humans and animals eat more than they need and build up fat tissues. Then, temperatures continuously drop until winter arrives. The earth lies still, leaves fall, and growth takes a rest. Only a limited amount of nonperishable foods, which continuously diminish during the winter months, are available to humans and animals. The caloric deficit is balanced by the body's reserves, primarily owing to our fat cells.

Just as nature comes out of hibernation and leaves and flowers unfold again in spring, humans can end their fast and gradually return to a regular diet, considered the »building-up« phase (see p. 100). This leads to a powerful reconstruction of new protein structures within nature and the human body, which is otherwise only known in children during periods of growth.

The ability to fast during food shortage, just like the ability to »over-eat« when there is a surplus of food, was the only chance for humans and animals to survive the irregularity of food supply on planet Earth. In animals, depending on the season and food availability, metabolism switches automatically from external nutrition to nutrition taken from fat reserves. Instinctively refusing food is not the

FROM MY EXPERIENCES

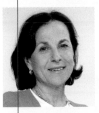

Why I Marvel at Penguins

The unbelievable length of their fast fascinates me: 6 months each year for about 35 years. The social behavior of fasting penguins fascinates me as well: in order to protect each individual against the icy storms, the entire penguin colony continuously rotates in a spiral pattern around itself, so that the animals on the outside slowly move to the center where the huddled bodies radiate ample heat—»instinctive altruism«! The king penguins protect each other from the cold: from −48°C on the outside, the temperature can rise up to +35°C at the center of the group! Humans could learn a thing or two from this type of solidarity. The entire being and appearance of penguins moves me. Maybe this is because they are so much like humans in the way they waddle along and caringly watch over the egg; not to speak of the drama that can unfold if the female cannot pass the egg fast enough to the male—the egg immediately freezes in the icy temperatures. This is much like a miscarriage.

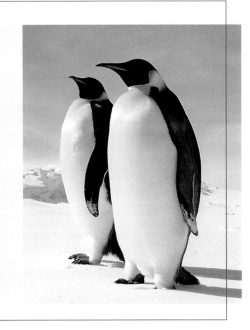

After this has been accomplished, the female passes the egg into the brood pouch of the lucky father and makes her way back to the ocean, where she rebuilds her body reserves. For more than 65 days, his fat belly serves the father-to-be as a nutritional storage chamber and the egg as protection against the cold (down to −40 to −50°C). Right before the fat reserves of the male are depleted, the chick hatches. The king penguin now restlessly awaits the return of the female. After 115 days of fasting, an irresistible signal urges him to return to the ocean to fish.

If the female returns in time to take over the chick, she feeds it with fish that she is able to preserve in her stomach for days. If the female does not return in time (e.g., she dies), the male leaves the chick, which cannot survive on its own. This shows the strength of the metabolic signal to rebuild his body reserves!

The metabolic rate at rest is reduced during the entire fast with the exception of the very first days. When the fat reserves are depleted to the extent that the bird's energy reserves are only sufficient to reach the ocean, those signals of the sympathetic nervous system that elevate the metabolic rate at rest increase: the penguin becomes restless, hyperactive—he must leave. Not only does the animal use up his remaining fat reserves on the walk back to the ocean, but also an increasing amount of protein. This protein breakdown is completely reversible if the penguin is back in time to eat.

Variable Feelings of Hunger

This signal—much like the signal for a fuel tank in a car switching to reserve—is also found when anorexic patients starve to death; unlike penguins anorexic individuals are unable to refeed. Physicians specializing in fasting in the past called this signal »true hunger«. It is perceived at the end of a fast lasting several weeks.

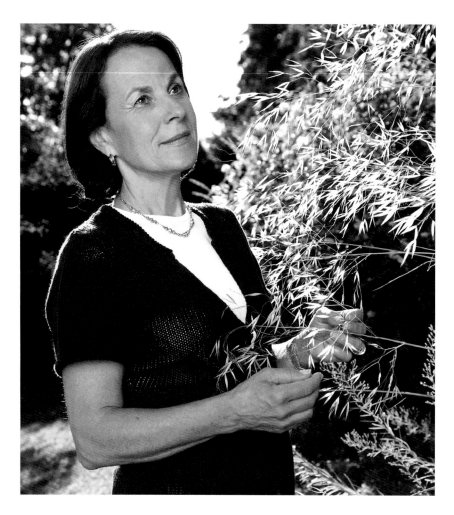

ence is craving and appetite, fueled by fantasizing about certain foods. These sensations rarely correspond to physical hunger.

During the first 3 days of fasting, before the metabolic switch is completed, feelings of hunger sometimes manifest themselves as an empty feeling or rumbling in the stomach, as well as through salivation. Afterward no hunger is felt anymore.

The Natural Yoyo Effect

Animals and humans who live in harmony with nature lose weight and regain the same weight depending on the season and food availability. This repeats itself every year. Variation in weight following the seasons is normal and can be considered a natural »yoyo effect.« In my opinion, obese humans who lose a lot of weight through random diets and regain uncontrolled amounts beyond their initial weight do not experience this natural yoyo effect. The king penguin fasts up to 6 months, going through different stages, its body weight varies accordingly and does so for 35 years on average. However, the penguin does not gain weight every year, but returns to its pre-fasting weight. The same happens in normal-weight people if they fast according to the method described in this book.

This »true hunger« is supposed to be an overwhelming sensation. In a person of normal weight fasting for more than 40 days, it generally »manifests itself with imperative force not only in the stomach but also through severe retching and swallowing reflex.« With these words, a former medical

specialist described this »signal« as a sign indicating the depletion of the reserves. (I have never observed this because shorter fasting periods are commonly practiced today.)

In the course of the fast, hunger ceases. What we sometimes experi-

Migratory Birds Fast

Birds are known to be the nomads of the skies and fly to places that provide them with food during the cold season. They must often travel for days without food and water. They utilize favorable air currents to save their body reserves, but on some stretches they depend entirely on their body reserves (fat, protein, micronutrients, and most of all water) for their athletic performance. They have the ability to condense their breath after expiration in their peaks and recycle it, in order to save water. On some stretches, swans travel at an altitude of 8000 m, at temperatures as low as −48°C to use their water reserve sparingly! A remarkable example of the art of fasting is the humming bird (*Archilochus colubris*). It weighs 5 g and uses 2 g of fat to travel non-stop more than 1000 km from New York across the Gulf of Mexico to Central America. For comparison, a small airplane consumes 800 L of kerosene on the same route.

A Mystery
Can you believe that migratory birds use protein from the muscles of their wings? You may reason that »it makes no sense for the bird to use protein from its wings—it must work with those wings.« Nevertheless, it is a known fact that during such a flight, a bird's wing and even the heart musculature diminishes, without decreasing its flight efficiency. This mystery is solved on page 34.

Women in Gambia

At a research station looking at metabolism in Gambia (West Africa), the British scientist Dr. Andrew Prentice studied a demographic group of humans who live very simply and in close contact with nature. He published a study about 20 000 women of child-bearing age whose weight was regularly controlled for 10 years. They weighed 53 kg on average and lost 5 kg every year during the monsoon season, when little food was available. This is considered a partial fast. On average, those women lost weight down to 48 kg and later regained what they had lost. These regular annual shifts in weight—similar to animals—did not show signs of being detrimental to health. Compared with continuously well-fed British women of the same age, the Gambian women were just as healthy and displayed fewer signs of osteoporosis, probably due to intense physical activity.

Today, we have scientific evidence showing that intermittent fasting and hypocaloric—but well-balanced—nutrition slows down aging processes.

Humans Can Fast as Well

» Humans can fast just like animals if there is a food shortage, for example, in winter or during the monsoon season. Humans developed the ability to store body reserves and mobilize them while fasting, out of the need to survive when they lacked food: fatty tissue is turned into energy. Vitamins, minerals, and essential fatty acids as well as some protein reserves are tapped into. Humans can choose to utilize the ability to live off their fat deposits at any time. Medical care in an appropriate environment is essential when the purpose of fasting is to prevent and treat diseases. Even when using this manual, it is advisable to be under competent care.

» Apparently, it is as difficult to deal with overabundance as it is to cope with deficiency.«
Dr. Heinz Fahrner

How I Discovered Fasting

Initially, I tried fasting for physical reasons. In my family there was a tendency to be overweight and as a child I was always chubby. In my teenage years, I was at odds with my weight and wanted to match the ideal of the slim beauty. I found a book about fasting and was fascinated. I thought to myself: »I must try this!«

I had my first fasting experience when I was 17. It was a revelation. During the fast I felt buoyant, sometimes euphoric, and wanted to change my whole life. I was in the midst of the separation process from a very strict home, which I perceived as confining. I was inspired by the spirit of 1968 and returning to my parent's home was like a rude awakening to reality. Nothing had changed there; all problems had remained the same.

In spite of the very difficult conditions I met with after my first fast, I was determined to repeat this experience. I wanted to be in charge of my eating habits. In a roundabout way I found out about the Buchinger clinic at Lake Constance in Überlingen. This is where I did my second fasting followed by further fasting visits.

One of my fasts at Überlingen was at the time when I prepared for my last medical finals. I kept to myself and had little or no contact with the other guests, because I wanted to study.

Every day I went to the public clinic library, where I felt very much at ease: I was usually by myself, surrounded by books, and had a marvelous view of

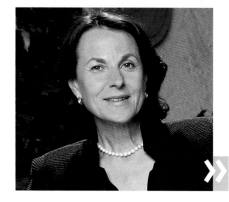

Lake Constance. One day I met a woman there who came from my home town of Geneva. She was well acquainted with my family. She was of an exuberant nature and as we were chatting, the words came simply pouring out of her: »I must introduce you to Raimund Wilhelmi, the junior director of the clinic. You have to marry him!«

I Met My Husband

I immediately felt attraction to Raimund Wilhelmi when I met him in person, but back then we lived in different worlds. He walked around in a suit and tie, because he was the junior director. I lived the 1968 way of life. My student friends

were nonconformists and wore beards. I returned home and passed my finals. Before starting my first position in the surgical ward of a clinic in Lausanne, I had the opportunity to cover for a member of staff of the Buchinger Clinic in Überlingen who was on vacation. During this period, I got to know my husband-to-be better. The stress over my finals was in the past and we became good friends. I was 28 and he was past 30. We realized quickly that »we had searched for a long time and finally found one another«; this is how we worded it in our wedding announcement. We felt that fate had brought us together and got married rather swiftly.

» Fasting has always been an important part of my life.

I finished my medical residency and began to work as a physician specializing in fasting at the Überlingen clinic.

My Mentors

One of my »mentors« was Dr. Heinz Fahrner, a great mind and systemic thinker in regard to fasting, who had worked as head physician at the clinic for 30 years. He regularly fasted—for preventive reasons and as a »metabolic workout«, because he was of the opinion that fasting trains many biochemical processes in the body. Today, some anti-aging techniques, for example, »dinner-cancelling« are based on the same concept. I was inspired by Dr.

Fahrner's holistic yet medically grounded perspective that separated fasting from esotericism and considered it a scientific method with great emphasis on the spiritual and humane component, an approach often lacking in medicine mostly taught at universities.

Another »mentor« was Dr. Catherine Kousmine, who researched the significance of nutrition in the treatment of cancer, MS, and polyarthritis. She gave me an understanding of the nutritional aspects. Early on, her intelligence, humor, and dedication to her profession steered my career toward integrative medicine.

Dr. Otto Buchinger

Dr. Otto Buchinger, my husband's grandfather, introduced me to the spiritual dimension of fasting. I basically devoured his books. Physical problems led him to discover fasting, as was the case with me. In 1917, he fell ill while he was a medical officer for the Imperial Navy. He developed rheumatic fever, a severe type of inflammation of the joints. In March 1918, at the age of 40, he had to be discharged from the Navy on total and permanent disability. Suffering greatly and physically handicapped, he followed a friend's advice to go for a therapeutic fast with Dr. Riedlin in Freiburg, Germany. »This 19-day cure truly saved my existence and my life. I was weak and thin, but I regained the ability to move my joints,« Buchinger wrote in his memoirs. Formerly disabled, he was now permanently cured,

healthy, and able to work again (which remained unchanged until his death at 89)! From here on, »the most powerful of all cures« determined Dr. Buchinger's professional path. In 1920, he admitted his first in-clinic fasting patients. As his success grew, the number of patients seeking help and healing grew; all expectations were exceeded and the hopes invested in fasting were fulfilled. Today, the therapeutic effects of fasting on joint diseases are scientifically documented.

Maria Buchinger

Born in 1916, Maria Buchinger was a close associate of her father and adopted all of Otto Buchinger's principles. Her

My husband and I fast regularly in our clinic.

recipe for youthfulness was: »Discipline, positive thinking, humor, no smoking, going to bed early, and a vegetarian diet.« She fasted regularly until the age of 86. Together with her husband Helmut Wilhelmi, who died in 1985, she founded the Buchinger Clinics in Überlingen, Germany and Marbella, Spain. Since that time, the management of the clinics has passed on to the third generation.

Maria Buchinger developed the humane dimension of fasting, which is the skill of guiding and caring for the fasting patients. The special »spirit« of the clinics in Überlingen and Marbella must be

ascribed to her: security, warm-heartedness, and attentiveness.

She respected the need for silence and solitude, but also brought people together who enriched each other. Her instinct never failed her.

The regular fasting cures that we participate in at our clinic are the milestones

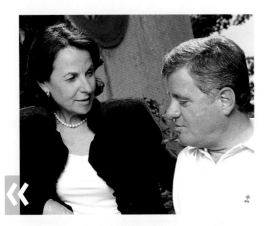

of my husband's and my life. On the following pages I will talk about some of these experiences. On page 46, my husband will give his explanation as to why he fasts on a regular basis.

With the help of our grown-up sons, Victor and Leonard, the Buchinger Clinics may arrive one day at the fourth generation. In the meantime, they appreciate the fasting periods at the clinic in Überlingen for being a time without cell-phones and Internet!

The Three Dimensions of Fasting

In many cultures fasting is viewed as a possibility to expand one's awareness, initiate readjustment processes, as well as a cleansing ritual.

Analogous to eating traditions, there are fasting traditions that have been strongly influenced by religion. Fasting is always linked to praying and »almsgiving«—three-dimensional fasting. In his book *Fasting: What? Why? How?*, the Jesuit priest Niklaus Brantschen offered a contemporary »translation« of the three dimensions:

1. Fasting, the medical–physical dimension, represents the physiological processes and the medical-therapeutic application.
2. Praying, the spiritual–religious dimension, results from the natural access to higher levels of consciousness during the fast, which is aspired to in all of the world religions.
3. »Almsgiving« (or charity, compassion), the socio-humane dimension, describes the heightened ability of a fasting person to be sensitive to those around them. It also refers to the group dynamics developing in a fasting community.

The holistic form of human fasting is voluntary fasting following medical guidelines, while perceiving the needs of fellow human beings, and being connected to the divine. In Christian tradition, fasting culminates in the Easter celebration, which symbolizes new life.

Religious fasting traditions generally neglected, or even punished the body. We owe it to physicians such as Dr. Otto Buchinger and his successors that medical care, in terms of a »physically beneficial asceticism« of the body during the fast was developed and applied for healing. In a later section, beginning on page 18, the medical–physical dimension ist dealt with. Dr. Buchinger's subsequent generations developed the Buchinger Amplius fasting method (see p. 88–89).

The Spiritual–Religious Dimension

» I deepened the spiritual dimension through repeated fasts in the Communauté de Grandchamp (on p. 13 I describe this in more detail), my friendship with Sister Christianne Méroz, and the writings of Dr. Otto Buchinger. In 1981, the nuns of the ecumenical Communauté de Grandchamp at Lake Neuchâtel in Switzerland wished to re-establish the traditional fasting procedure, including contemporary medical adjustments. Since 1981, I have regularly fasted with them and provided medical counsel to a fasting group comprising nuns and their guests. The religious message is: fasting does not only serve oneself, one's health and beauty, it also addresses »the other«; the same is true whether fasting in a group or alone. Religious fasting rituals and rules wish to save humans from egocentric, show-oriented renouncements, the motto being:

» But when you fast, anoint your head and wash your face that your fasting may not be seen by others but by your Father who is in secret. And your Father who sees in secret will reward you.«

Matthew 6, 17–18 (English Standard Version)

Mahatma Gandhi is a great figure in Indian history. There were two important aspects of his faith: non-violence and fasting. His fasting periods, lasting several weeks, have become famous in context with Indian independence and served the renewal of his spiritual powers. His fasts had nothing to do with hunger strikes but were a physical form of prayer.

» What the eyes are for the outer world, fasts are for the inner.«

Gandhi

Today, fasting for peaceful relations, according to Gandhi's example, is practiced by various groups. For example, in the Communauté de l'Arche, founded by Lanza del Vasto in France, two members who are at odds with each other fast until their conflict is resolved.

Ramadan

The three pillars of the Judeo-Christian fasting tradition (fasting, praying, and almsgiving) are complemented by two additional pillars in the Islamic tradition: the Creed and the pilgrimage to Mecca.

◀ Following Augustinus, Niklaus Brantschen, Swiss Jesuit, writes: »Prayer and active charity are the two wings of fasting without which it cannot lift off.«

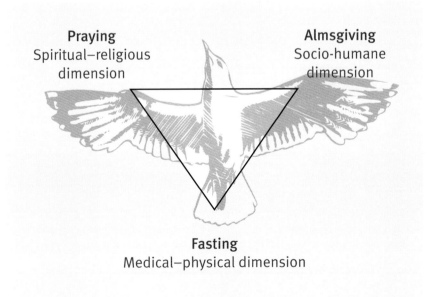

Praying
Spiritual–religious dimension

Almsgiving
Socio-humane dimension

Fasting
Medical–physical dimension

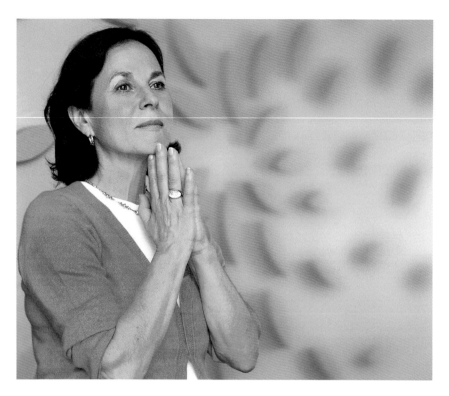

People become tired and gain weight, instead of gaining clarity and sereneness. When traditions lose their context and meaning, they are at risk of disappearing, as has happened to the Christian fasting tradition.

Yom Kippur

The Jewish people must dedicate 10 days, between the Jewish New Year and the Day of Atonement (Yom Kippur) to repentance (Teshuvah) and reflection. In the final 24 hours of this period, the day of Yom Kippur, no one drinks or eats and everyone prays at the synagogue.

For one month, between sunrise and sunset, neither food nor water is allowed to be consumed during »Ramadan,« the Islamic fasting season. The socio-humane dimension is especially cultivated; every day the entire family gathers for prayer. Once a day, after sunset, a modest ritual fasting meal is eaten, and one place at the table is reserved for a poor person. In today's world this, as well as other useful traditions, is not always adhered to. Worries about scarcity, and the pleasure of eating, may lead to lavish meals that last the entire night. Unfortunately, this prevents the bare essentials from taking place, the switching on of the fasting metabolism.

The Socio-Humane Dimension

» What does »almsgiving« mean to you? In a literal sense, it probably means donating money for a good cause. An Early Christian book of wisdom teaches us: »The one who has nothing to give, shall fast and give his brothers what he would have spent that day.«

Almsgiving does not only mean to share one's abundance, it can mean something like »appreciation of others.« Fasting humans, just like fasting penguins (see p. 4), tend to support each other and treat each other with more tolerance. Social barriers break down and people return to a state of existential equality. The potential for aggression decreases in a fasting group, emotions are less repressed, and people open up and communicate more freely. It is not uncommon for lasting relations to begin here.

»Abstention creates awareness for the need of others,« Lanza del Vasto states. Living in industrialized countries, we know that we can return to eating after the fast, but we may gain insight into the world of hunger.

My Soul Food

In the past 40 years, during which I returned to my actual faith and to the spiritual dimension of life, I realized how frequently fasting is mentioned in books of wisdom, particularly the Bible. The biblical fasting descriptions are a source of inspiration to me.

I come from the Judeo-Christian tradition and participate in the development of globalized ethics. I stick to my tradition but I am open to all other forms of spirituality. The Bible mentions numerous famous fasts:

- The fast of David recognizing his crime, expanding awareness, and returning to God (II Samuel 12, 16–23).
- The three-day fast of Esther that enabled her in all her beauty and presence to ask the King, her husband, for the salvation of her people—and it was granted to her (Esther 4, 16–17).
- The fast of Elias and Moses—40 days and nights—to meet with God on top of the mountain. There, Moses received the Ten Commandments (Exodus 34, 28).
- The fast of Jesus that prepared him for his mission (Lucas 4, 2).

Communauté de Grandchamp

When fasting in the Communauté de Grandchamp, the sorority invites us to meet with them in the chapel five times a day. The rhythm of the prayers is like a heartbeat. This is where I experience security and connection to myself, the community, and the world. Once each day, everyone shares how he or she is doing (*partage*).

Was anything special experienced, wondering or amazement, insights for oneself? Was there a difficulty, crisis, or a moment of discouragement? These moments of awareness are shared with all the members of the group. In the Communauté de Grandchamp, I have learned how to fast for someone else, like dedicating a prayer to someone. The nuns, for example, fast for those in need, a nation at war or threatened by famine.

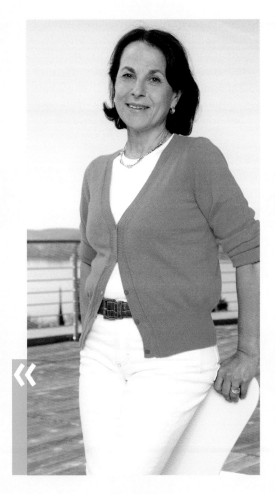

What I am seeking nowadays during my fasts is serenity, harmony between body and soul, and being in the present. From a place of calmness that lies deep within, we can view everything with amazement. We are focused inwardly.

Spirituality and Fasting

Spirituality begins with having time—you have time when you are fasting. Spirituality means allowing things to happen. The body is allowed to mobilize the stored nutrients as needed during the fast, without active control of the mind. Spirituality means to be present here and now, and to accept what comes about.

Quietness is part of the spiritual fasting experience, also giving access to the inner silence. Chatting, gossiping, and judging should be avoided. This is facilitated by the particular repose that settles into the body. The power plant of nutrition and metabolism, including its syntheses, transport of nutrients, production of juices, and gastrointestinal motion, does not rule the daily rhythm any longer, but is shut down. Harmonious moods and feelings of happiness often develop (see p. 36). All behavioral patterns are interrupted during the fast. Like performing a quantum leap, a new space of time is entered. It is a spiritual challenge to affirm this empty space and trust its emergence. The spiritual dimension unfolds in this space.

What Nourishes Our Souls?

» In everyday life, the hunger of the soul is often mistaken for the need for food. The fast offers the opportunity to attend to one's own spiritual needs, which become more transparent.

» During the fast the body thrives, but the soul starves.«

Dr. Otto Buchinger

In his book *Guidelines for Taking Care of Your Soul (Die Hygiene des inneren Menschen)* Dr. Otto Buchinger listed nine elements that were important to him and that are able to nourish a person's soul—not only during the fast but always. He called them the »nutrition of the soul.« The wording of his reflections dating from 1947 may sound a little antiquated but to me the content is important and essential. I would like to interpret and comment on it from my contemporary point of view.

1. Fulfilling Work

»Plentiful, meaningful, regulated, dutiful, and enjoyable work including appropriate breaks.«

Yes, how I feel about my work, my occupation, is important. Do I approve of what I do? Do I find meaning in my work? Does it fulfill me? There will be plenty of joyous moments in my life if I can identify with my work and not simply look forward to my leisure time. Happy people (according to today's happiness research) are truly involved with their occupation without being over-worked.

2. Reading

»The spiritually animated person, who always strives to thrive, must read.«

I feel the same way. I especially enjoy reading during a fast. Reading requires time and an inner openness, so that what I read has the space to resonate.

▶ While fasting, I am more inclined to take the time and get thoroughly involved in a book.

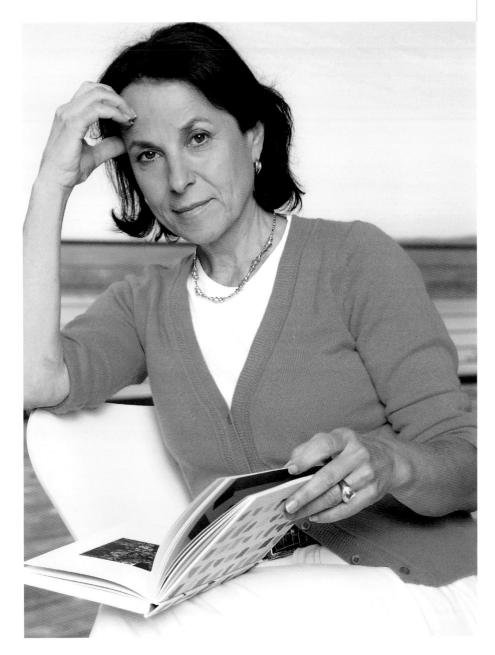

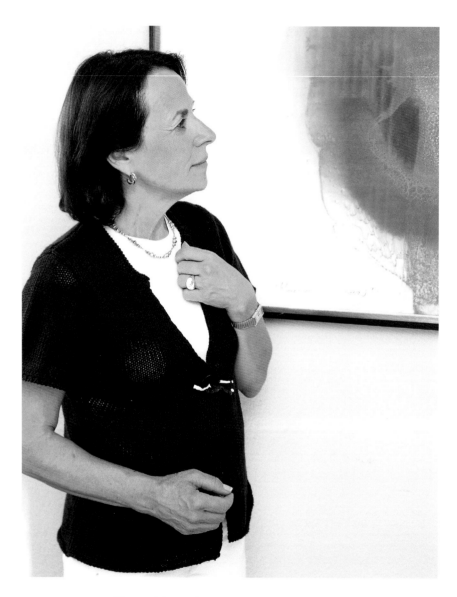

▲ It can be truly »nourishing« to be completely rapt in contemplation of a picture.

The text communicates with my experiences, my associative world, and enriches it.

3. Good Companions

»I do believe that humans have invisible companions. In addition, each of us has a guardian angel. How do I find good companions? Answer: using the adequate decoy for these beings, spiritual food: memorized proverbs, mantras, quick prayers, one's own poignant observations, apt lyrical passages, verse from psalms and hymns, suitable quotations from dramas, passages from dramatic monologues, and stanzas from fervent chants.«

I think of synchronicities, the unbelievable so-called coincidences in life, helpful encounters that were most unlikely and took place anyway, just like my chance meeting in the library (p. 8). The idea of angels being at work sounds quite poetic to me. Otto Buchinger called synchronicities signatures. The idea that angels can be enticed and attracted sounds motivating! The more I wish for an angel or a sign, the more I pay attention, the more numerous is their appearance because I am open to perceiving them.

4. Nature

»Nature: it's a spa. Let us walk and wander about more often!«

When I'm hiking or in-line skating, or back when I used to ski, nature is and was a source of energy and joy to me. Particularly during a fast, I contemplate nature. I must be outdoors every day, no matter the weather! I love gardens. Gardens provide activity in fresh air and admiration for their beauty, which is simply for its own sake.

5. Music

»The rhythm, the sound, and the melody always affect man and beast (who knows, maybe they also affect the sensitive plants), change moods, and act on body and soul.«

When fasting I flee the constant background music and look forward to music that I carefully choose and celebrate. It amplifies the inner quietness. Sometimes I sing. To me, all of this is an act of connecting and being present; listening attentively—to the music and the emotions that arise.

6. Graphic Art Appreciation

»What greets us from the walls is part of our soul food.«

We exhibit contemporary art on the walls of our clinics and offer our guests an art studio that allows them to be creative: painting, or modeling something. Our collection of art and our corporate identity are colorful, bright, and contemporary. Every human carries a virtual museum within, storing all pictures, some of which arise in association with current situations.

7. Humor

»The God-given blessing of a character trait. Is it inborn? Does one possess it? Or is it missing completely sometimes? Can one acquire it or can it be taught? Blessed is the one who possesses it, because it is the healthiest outfit of the soul.«

I cherish the ability to laugh about myself, especially about repetitive behavior patterns or my ego forcing me into complaints and dramas. I become serene and light-hearted during the fast. It may come as a surprise to fasting skeptics, but there is much laughter in a fasting clinic.

8. Volunteering

»Naturally, this refers to serving mankind.«

Volunteering brings us back to the idea of almsgiving, which pertains to fasting in all religions. During a fast, people open up to each other. They give their time, attention, and sometimes money for certain projects. This is not about giving to be a better person, but about selfless acts that bring joy to all concerned.

9. Meditation

»›Meditation‹ and ›adoration‹; reflection about the meaning of life and ›worshipping‹.«

Meditation primarily means presence and recess of mental activity to me. It means to employ all senses to perceive people, places, and situations without judging, labeling, or criticizing right away; exercising life here and now, feeling alive through every cell of the body. Owing in part to our former head of medicine, Dr. Christian Kuhn, who introduced the quietness of Zen meditation to our clinic, we create a spiritual atmosphere in our clinic. After retiring from my administrative office, I would like to offer group meditations together with Dr. Kuhn and create spaces where people can practice letting go. Through my own religious tradition, I am well acquainted with prayer and the inner dialogue.

It may be easier to forgo material indulgence or addictions, like over-eating, smoking, drinking alcohol, if we manage to introduce these nine elements of soul food to our lives.

What Happens in Our Body when We Fast?

You will now find out more about the physiological background of fasting; what happens in your body while you temporarily give up external nutrition. What nutrition does for a person eating, the stored reserves do for a person fasting.

Why do we need nutrition?

- Nutrition is the fuel (primarily fat and carbohydrate) for our metabolism, generating energy and heat.
- Nutrition provides the building blocks (proteins, carbohydrates, essential fats, and minerals) for growth in children and for the renewal of body cells and structures in adults.

- Nutrition (especially fresh and natural food) provides bioactive substances (vitamins, minerals, secondary plant compounds also called phytoprotectants) that are the building blocks and fuels ensuring all vital functions.
- Food tastes good, is enjoyable, and brings people together. It is part of social life and culture to gather at the table.

The Two Nutritional Programs

» The word »eating« is usually associated with ingesting something tasty. It actually means to supply our body cells with nutrition. This is ensured in two ways, hence two nutritional programs exist:
  - Eating or nutritional program I, where food is ingested, is processed by the digestive system, and nourishes the body cells.

- Fasting or nutritional program II, where the digestive tract is at rest and the body cells receive predigested nutrition from the body's storage, primarily fat tissue.

Humans and animals can easily switch from one program to the other, especially if they regularly practice fasting or sports.

Program I—Eating

This is the normal situation. We nourish ourselves through eating and drinking, generally three times a day. The entire digestive tract, from the oral cavity to the rectum, breaks down and processes the food. The usable micro- and macronutrients are transported to the body cells via the blood:

- Digestion creates and radiates heat while supplying us with energy and nutritional building blocks.
- The building blocks that are delivered to the cells aid growth and replace old or damaged components.
- Hunger and satiety control food intake. The two hormones leptin and ghrelin play their regulating part in the background. However, many people do not eat according to the body's signals, particularly when sweet and fatty foods are available, but follow their cravings for pleasure. They are in danger of consuming more than their cells require and gaining weight. At this point, they are under the influence of the hormonal reward system of dopamine.
- Humans possess great energetic capacities. On demand, they can accelerate and produce maximum performance, but eating excessively decreases the performance.

▶ In everyday life, we drink a cup of tea in passing. During a fast, drinking a cup of tea is celebrated.

Program II—Fasting

- During a fast, no food is ingested and the body switches to »internal nutrition« for some time.
- The energy sources come from the body's deposits (fat tissue and some protein structures), without the involvement of the digestive tract. The radiating heat that is produced during digestion subsides.
- The body's reserves, mobilized from its tissues, are used for cell renewal and growth.

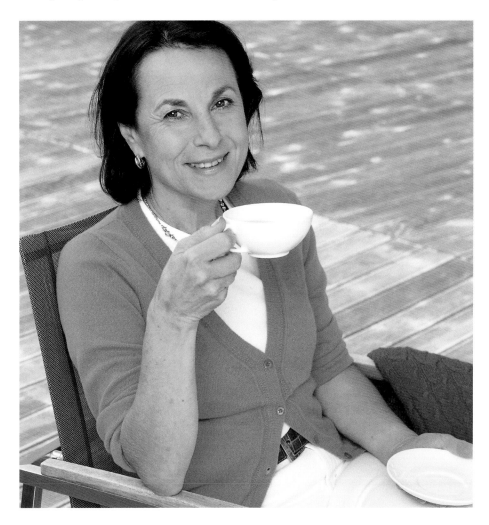

19

- The autopilot frugality sets in. There is no hunger and no satiety; a very special state.
- We can maintain an adequate energy level, as long as stress and acceleration are avoided and the pace of life is deliberate and reduced.

Fuel Supply

Humans function just like cars: no fuel, no movement. Human fuels—when eating—are carbohydrates (glucose) and fats. If the food intake is higher than required, the body builds up fat pads, comparable to the fuel spare can in the car. When fasting, the fat cells pass the stored calories on to the blood, which ensures continuous nourishment of the entire body, just from within. In terms of the car example, the driver would not go to a gas station but use the spare cans.

This example is to illustrate that fasting does not mean lack of nutrition but switching to stored nutrition. During a fast, we are still continuously supplied with fuel. A second example will clarify this even more. When you work with your laptop, you initially plug it into an electrical outlet. From there, it is supplied with electricity and at the same time its battery is charged. When you pull the plug, the charged battery will supply the energy. The greater the charge

capacity of the battery, the longer you can use the laptop without direct power connection.

How Long Do the Fat Reserves Last?

Overweight people have a greater »fat battery« than normal-weight people, hence they can fast longer. The reserves of normal-weight adults last approximately 40 days, reserves of overweight people last longer.

The »menu« of a fasting normal-weight person includes:
- ca. 0.75 kg carbohydrates (glycogen);
- ca. 3 kg protein; and
- ca. 10 kg fat.
When utilizing ca. 2500 kcal a day, this equates to approximately 40 days.

With 20 kg overweight, the »menu« of the fasting person approximately includes:

Both nutritional programs supply us with the necessary energy and building blocks for cell renewal. Both nutritional programs can produce well-being and contentment, if executed properly. How does the switching from I to II actually work?

- 1.25 kg carbohydrates (glycogen);
- ca. 4 kg protein; and
- ca. 25 kg fat.

This would allow fasting for 100 days (according to Cahill). These numbers represent theory. A fast under medical supervision generally lasts 1 to 3 weeks and in rare cases up to 40 days.

Energy for the Brain

When forgoing eating, one's »fasting program« starts up quickly and taps into the fat reserves. This could lead to the conclusion that one comfortably utilizes the fat reserves until the fast is ended. This would mean, at least for industrialized countries, people can fast without the least problem.

It is not quite that simple. Fat supplies most body tissues with energy, but one main system, the central nervous system, including the brain, requires sugar (glucose) for fuel. It takes a few days until the nervous system switches to burning fat.

How is the glucose supply to the brain ensured during the first days of a fast?
- A small amount of natural glucose is supplied by the supplements (juices, honey).
- The glycogen storage in the liver can supply the brain for one day.

20

▶ When the transition phase has passed I feel light and happy.

▬ Fat cannot be transformed into glucose, but protein can. This is called gluconeogenesis (glucose renewal). Especially during the first days of a fast, minor amounts of protein building blocks (amino acids) are released from the proper structures (see figure on p. 33) and are transformed into glucose for the brain.

What does the energy supply for the brain look like during the further course of the fast?

▬ During the course of the fast, the brain adapts to the utilization of fat in the form of ketone bodies. The majority of energy generated during the fast originates from fat burning.
▬ When fat deposits are broken down, glycerol molecules are released, which can then be transformed into glucose. This is another way to supply the brain with energy.
▬ Protein mobilization for gluconeogenesis is reduced to a minimum.

An explosive reconstruction of protein structures takes place when returning to ingesting food. Also during the fast, protein synthesis continues to take place via recycled proteins: hair and nails still grow and old skin cells are shed and replaced by new

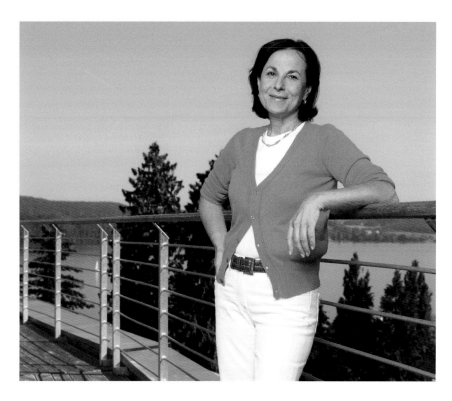

ones. The cells of the intestinal mucous membranes are subject to »autodigestion« and are newly synthesized at once during the building-up phase.

»Building Block« Supply

Protein is required for cell renewal during a fast. I would like to explain this phenomenon. Humans are born weighing approximately 3.5 kg. In order to grow up into a normal-weight adult, they have to gain 15 to 20 times this weight. After that growth is completed and humans are »grown up«, nutriments now deliver the »building blocks« for the renewal of bodily structures. All body tissues are continuously renewed: every second, thousands of cells die and are replaced by new ones. Mucous mem-

21

branes and skin cells are renewed in a few days, bone cells in a few months. The body may be compared with a house that is initially built with a lot of different materials and later is regularly maintained and renovated (wallpaper and carpets sooner than roof and walls).

Vitamins and Minerals

Humans possess stores of many vitamins (e.g., A and B12) for months and years. Vitamins and minerals are utilized sparingly. Because the metabolism works more efficiently during a fast, the majority of the digestive processes are no longer required, which signifies considerable conservation of vitamins and minerals (e.g., to produce digestive juices, to process nutrients and cross membranes to transport them to the cells). Humans use their body's own »ready-to-use products«! Humans and animals do not require vitamin and mineral supplements when they live naturally and have had an adequate nutritional supply before they fast (also see p. 79).

Switching to »Autopilot«

Can you deliberately slow down your pulse rate or stop digestion? No. Some functions of the human body are beyond the control of the mind but are regulated by the autonomic nervous system as well as hormones, for example, respiration, digestion, heart rate, and also the metabolism while fasting. In a sense, they run on »autopilot« and are controlled by sympathetic (acceleration) and parasympathetic systems (deceleration).

Sympathetic System
At the beginning of a fast, adrenaline, a sympathetic neurotransmitter, dominates the system. It is released when blood sugar levels drop and the stomach is empty. Adrenaline sends an alarm signal to the metabolism: »Shift! There is no more external nutrition. Get sugar reserves from the liver (glycogen). Fat cells, you get ready to release fatty acids. Liver, sustain us through your protein storage. To all tissues in the body: release your dispensable proteins and water!« This adrenergically mediated prompt is replaced or intensified by other hormones (glucagon, growth hormones, and thyroid hormones). The sympathetic system demands that mouth, stomach, and intestines reduce their juice production and activities; at the same time, it demands a stronger heartbeat. The production of cortisone is also stimulated during this initial stage, and expresses its anti-inflammatory properties.

Parasympathetic System
Approximately 3 days after these sympathetic encouragements, the transition into the parasympathetic stage takes over. The calmer waters of the fasting metabolism have been reached:
- Blood pressure (when elevated) drops to normal levels.
- Pulse rate slows down.
- Blood sugar levels out at low standard value.
- Fat cells continuously release fat from their stores. This fat is transformed into ketone bodies and releases its glycerol portion.

The production of thyroid hormones decreases because fasting is tied to energy conservation. The digestive tract enjoys a break and the chance for a clean-up. In order to spare cell proteins, the growth hormone slows down protein mobilization while glucose is not ingested. The hormone aldosterone regulates the hydration balance. Ultimately, the fasting person will dress a little warmer, because he/she lacks the heat that is normally generated through digestion.

Autopilot— What Does it Feel Like?

I call this stage autopilot because we are not subject to the system of hunger and satiety any longer. We reach a permanent state of not-being-hungry, nor do we feel satieted as satiety goes hand in hand with the fullness originating in the gastrointestinal tract.

Now instead of entering the body via the digestive system, where it is processed and assimilated, nutrition comes directly from the fat cells releasing fat into the blood stream. The digestive system is shut down with the exception of its basic functions.

In some people, the change from nutritional program I (nutrition from the outside) to nutritional program II (nutrition from the inside) is almost imperceptible. Other people experience noticeable adjustments. Athletic, young, or energetic people feel the least affected. The same may be true for people who are experienced in fasting.

During the Adjustment I Feel Listless

The adjustment (adaptation stage) lasts 2 to 3 days. During this time most people initially experience some sort of restlessness, do not sleep well, and have intense dreams. During the day these people feel tired, their blood pressure drops, and they may feel listless. I regularly experience this state as my blood pressure is generally low and I am usually under job-related stress before I start fasting. I fall into a state of fatigue and feel like a bear that wants to hibernate away from it all.

The adjustment is not easy for me because of this leaden weariness. In the beginning I lie down and sleep a lot. I accept this condition and do not fight it. The adaptation stage can also bring on a headache, which I am not affected by at all. Heartburn or nausea may also occur because it takes a while for the digestive system to slow down.

I Live From Within Myself

A whole new energy level is reached when the adaptation stage has passed. The autopilot is turned on, which always feels like a miracle to me. I enter the space of internal tranquility. My room is suddenly organized, I have time, and energy is immediately available. I yield to the day–night rhythm, going to bed early (10 p.m.) and waking up early. After a few days I need less sleep and frequently wake up well rested at 5 a.m.

While on autopilot the nutrition of the cells is a calm and unobtrusive process as ingestion and digestive motion are absent. The body feels amazingly quiet inside, the abdomen becomes flat. There is no more fatigue after a meal! The energy that was required for digestion is now put to use for body cleansing.

»Deceleration«

The autopilot does not provide energy for acceleration but for consistent long-term utilization. When I forget something, I do not turn around and run to get it. That would not do me any good. One is forced to adapt a slow and intense rhythm.

This slower way of life brings about more respect for myself and for everyone around me. I become more conscious of the things I do, say, and experience. In general, I am quiet more often.

The Effects of Fasting

»Why are you fasting? You are not over-weight!« This quotation demonstrates how little information many of our contemporaries have about the range of therapeutic effects of fasting—other than weight reduction. It is a plausible fact that fat is reduced during a fast. But how can an inflamed knee joint, hay fever, or a migraine become alleviated? I will explain it to you.

In industrialized countries, many disorders are caused by over-eating or bad eating habits. Many measured values normalize during fasting. They include fat, cholesterol, triglycerides, sugar, and insulin. Pathological proteins, water, and toxic substances are eliminated.

After ridding metabolically active, internal surfaces of metabolic debris and deposits, cell and organ functions, as well as immune functions, improve and cell renewal is stimulated.

》 Fasting is the strongest appeal to the natural self-healing power of humans, physically and spiritually.«

Dr. Heinz Fahrner

Dr. Jürgen Rhode, retired chief of medicine of a clinic for integrative medicine in Berlin, Germany, conducted a vitality test recognized by gerontologists and proved the follow-

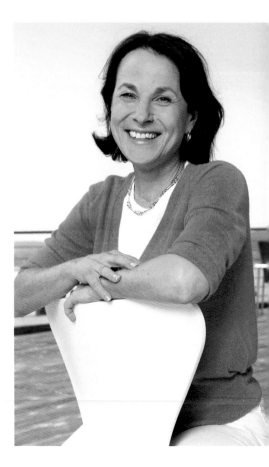

ing: after a 3-week in-patient fast, a rejuvenation effect and a reduction of the biological age of up to 6 years was noted.

The cleansed body, increased performance, reduced weight, improved blood flow properties, improved macro- and micro-circulation, and harmonized mood, are direct effects of fasting combined with improved quality of life and vitality. For some people, this becomes even more noticeable when protein synthesis is boosted after the fast.

What are the Primary Effects?

I would like to analyze the primary effects for you and illustrate how fasting is beneficial in metabolic and chronic inflammatory disorders. The table on page 26 offers a summary of the effects of fasting, in terms of indications and possible side-effects. The following text will elucidate the individual effects in more detail.

Fat and Insulin Reduction
Your body mobilizes its fat reserves when you deliberately stop eating. The blood is »skimmed« if it contains excessive fat. Triglycerides drop rapidly and the cholesterol count normalizes. A fatty liver will also release its excess fat. Fat deposits within the abdominal cavity and around the face and neck reduce especially quickly. The typical female deposits around the hips, thighs, and buttocks reduce more slowly (as they serve as reserves in case of pregnancy and breast-feeding). The weight loss in overweight people is quite obvious.

Blood sugar levels drop and as a result, insulin production decreases. In overweight diabetics, blood test results often normalize drastically during a fast. Dietary and lifestyle changes are required to maintain these results. Otherwise, the count will rise again quickly after the fast.

KNOWLEDGE

What Does Detoxification (Detox) Mean?

How can fasting contribute to detox if a person does not take in additional quantities of nutrients?
The term detoxification or »*Entschlackung*« is a metaphor conceived by Dr. Otto Buchinger. On the one hand it refers to a subjective feeling of well-being, the lightness and increasing clarity experienced by the person fasting. On the other hand it applies to objective bodily changes: cleansed skin, improved breathing, and reduction of complaints.
Detoxification of certain substances, found in excessive quantities in the blood, is additionally achieved, for example, cholesterol, other fats in the blood, glucose, too high storages of fats, and plaques of arteriosclerosis on the walls of arteries. Certain disease-causing AGEs—advanced glycation end products—or immune complexes are also reduced. Fasting mostly normalizes blood counts and reduces fat deposits. At the same time, typical arterial sclerotic deposits are reduced when consuming foods that are nearly fat-free. The same is to be expected from fasting. The tendency for protein utilization during fasting makes it plausible that degenerated or pathological protein structures are »self digested.«

Effects of fasting: indications and possible side-effects

Primary effects	Therapeutic effects on some indications	Possible side-effects
Fat and insulin reduction Glucagon and growth hormone ↑	▪ Overweight (excessive fat in the deposits) ↓ ▪ Hyperlipidemia (excessive fat in the blood) ↓ ▪ Fatty liver (excessive fat in the liver) ↓ ▪ Diabetes mellitus type II (excessive glucose in the blood) ↓ ▪ Arteriosclerosis ↓	▪ Acidoketosis ▪ Gout attack ▪ Hypoglycemia
Quieting of the gastrointestinal tract, cessation of antigen contact, modulation of the immune response, reduction of inflammatory processes	▪ Chronic diseases of the digestive tract (stomach, intestines, liver, pancreas, gallbladder) ▪ Immune deficiencies, allergies ↓ ▪ Polyarthritis (rheumatoid arthritis), joint disorders, and other chronic inflammatory diseases ↓	▪ Relapse of symptoms when food is re-introduced too quickly during the building-up phase
Water and salt elimination	▪ Hypertension ↓ ▪ Circulatory disorders (venous and arterial) ↓ ▪ Edema ↓	▪ Blood pressure is too low ▪ Mineral imbalance
Protein utilization (intra- and extracellular)	▪ »Rejuvenation« of the protein pool during the building-up phase ↑ ▪ Modulation of the immune system ▪ Improved exchange of gases and nutrients between cells and vessels	▪ When fasting for several weeks, loss of fat-free mass
Neurovegetative switch Hormonal changes	▪ Following a brief stressful period in the beginning: normalization of blood pressure and pulse rate, lowering of stress, calming down ▪ Neurohormonal »reset«	
Increased effects of serotonin Antidepressive, anxiolytic, and harmonizing effects	▪ Depressed moods ↓ ▪ Listlessness ↓	▪ Unconscious abuse of fasting as »endogenous doping,« e.g., anorexia nervosa
Antithrombotic effect	▪ Risk of thrombosis ↓	▪ Bleeding when medication is continued (anticoagulation)
Aversion to smoking Breaking of behavior patterns	▪ Smoking ↓	

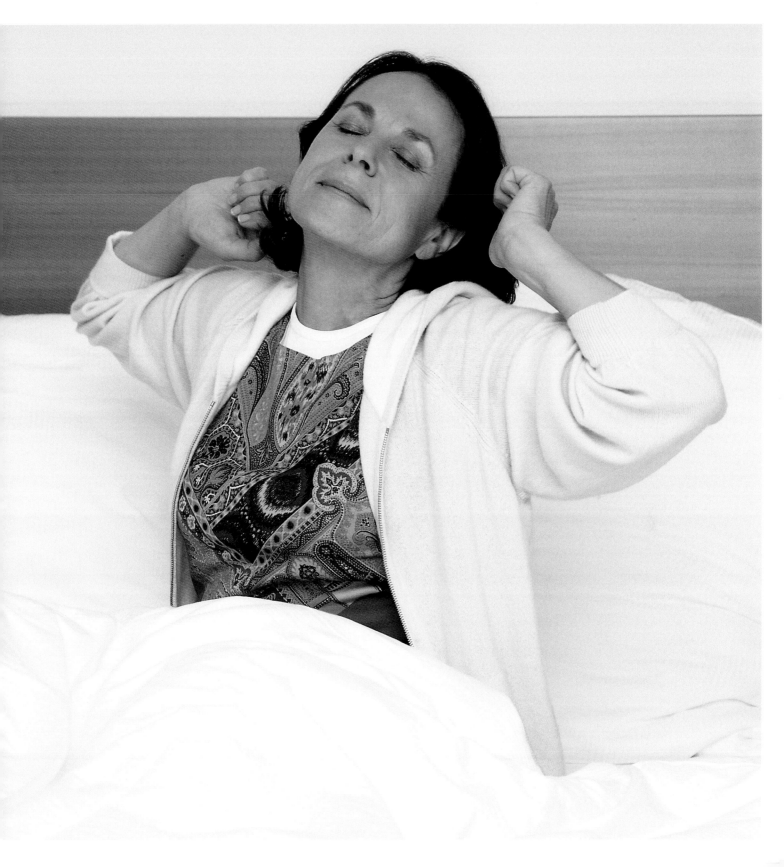

Losing Weight

You will lose weight when fasting. Women lose an average of 200 to 500 g per day and men slightly more. It is best to be under the therapeutic care of a physician, to exercise daily, and be looked after by a nutritionist and a physical therapist when treating an overweight (more than 25 kg/m² body mass index) condition.

The primary significance of fasting in association with fighting overweight is to acquire the ability to maintain the reduced weight and not only to lose the most weight possible per day. The Buchinger Amplius fasting program offers movement, relaxation, and health training, which supports patients in finding different eating and behavior patterns after the fast. Also, the Buchinger Amplius fasting program offers the opportunity to evaluate one's personal situation and find new emotional balance. The overweight person is assisted in replacing eating for pleasure without nutritional need and in compensating negative emotions with »soul food.«

In institutions concerned with fasting the following observations have been made:

- In cases of moderate overweight (frequently associated with risk factors for cardiovascular disease), fasting can reduce weight and protect against further weight gain, especially when fasting is repeated once a year.
- In cases of severe overweight, positive and lasting results are achieved through in-patient fasts in three to four stages.

Why are Many People Overweight these Days?

I am convinced that the individual is not solely responsible for being overweight. There are a number of components:

- The first component is hedonism, pleasure in eating. People want to be free to eat what tastes good to them. Usually, sweet and fatty tastes good. Many people utilize food for compensation and to rebalance their emotions. Others do the same using alcohol, drugs, and smoking, which are even more harmful.
- The second component is our so-called »toxic environment.« We are only partly responsible for barely exercising our bodies. Machines take care of everything. Everything is so fast-paced. Few people would appreciate that we arrived late because we decided to walk. In addition, food is omnipresent. We have access to food at all times and it always tastes delicious thanks to the »food design« invented by the food industry.
- The third component is the secondary results of the fast-paced lifestyle, including permanent stress, hectic

lives, and lack of time for enjoyment. I do not believe that it is helpful to measure the success of fasting only in weight reduction! What if an overweight fasting person does not attain the ideal weight right away? There are other positive effects to be accomplished, such as calming down, working through issues, and discovering new sources of pleasure besides eating and drinking.

Successful Fasting

I often think of a female patient who so far has »only« been able to reduce her weight from 130 kg down to 110 kg. But she has made huge progress regarding her autonomy. She moved out of her parents' home, got married, and wishes for a child. Her fasting has been successful. After five years she finally made the »breakthrough« to less than 80 kg. Experience has shown that long-term overweight is more persistent than recently and quickly gained weight, for example, during or after a pregnancy or when one quits smoking and starts eating sweets instead. One patient had gained 20 kg through her pregnancy and permanently lost it again by fasting once.

Another 40-year-old female patient ate out of frustration and despair and ended up weighing 82 kg. She fasted for 26 days and left us weighing 71 kg. Her abdominal girth was reduced from 86 to 81 cm. Fasting, the associated psycho-therapy, and relaxation exercises helped her to overcome her depression and discontinue her antidepressants. Fasting is

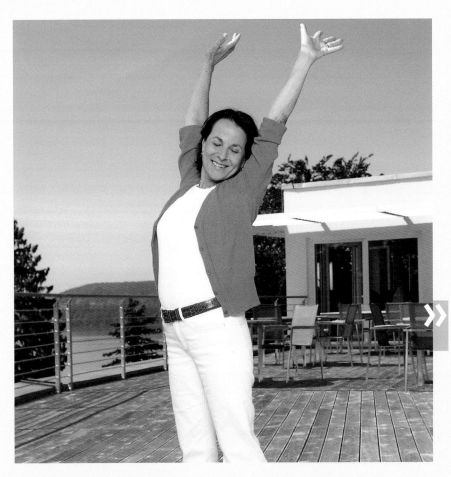

Will Weight be Regained after Fasting?

People who consume a lot of »junk food« and alcohol and exercise little, and who return to their old lifestyle after the fast, generally regain weight in excess of their initial weight. This is true regardless of whether the weight was lost by fasting, diets, or other methods. Determinants in terms of maintaining a lowered weight are lifestyle changes regarding nutrition and exercise, as well as aspiring emotional balance without compensation through food or alcohol. These means of compensation could be replaced by the soul foods that I listed on pages 14–17.

» Even though I am not overweight, I like to see the little fat pads of the tummy melt away during the fast.

Statistics from the Buchinger Clinic at Lake Constance are generated through data gathered from patients who have fasted at least 10 times (once a year as traditionally recommended):

- One-third of the subjects weighed less than at the beginning of their first fast.
- One-third weighed approximately the same as they did before their first fast despite increasing age.
- One-third gained weight despite regular fasts. The weight gain was not overwhelming.

especially suitable in treating reactive depression, that is, a persistent depressive mood caused by a life crisis that must be dealt with. When this patient returned home, she continued to reduce her weight and exercise regularly. The following year she came back to the clinic with the aim of reaching her ideal weight and stabilizing her condition. During this second fast she reduced her

weight from 70 down to 63 kg (1.70 m height).

For most people it is not difficult to maintain their weight for 6 months after the fast. But when Christmas season arrives, or sooner, the new eating pattern is undermined. Another fast should follow when the weight is supposed to drop further or when a new weight gain is noted.

Arteriosclerosis

The American doctor Dean Ornish achieved the regression of deposits in the arteries (arteriosclerosis) and an improvement of cardiovascular disorders through a rigorous low-fat diet, exercise, and meditation.

Presumably, the total lack of fat during fasting, accompanied by exercise and meditation has the same effects.

A Break for Digestion

The digestive canal is a unit composed of oral cavity, esophagus, stomach, small intestine, large intestine, and rectum. Ingested food is reduced to small pieces and processed, with the result that its nutrients can be

type II, stress, lack of exercise, and smoking.

heartburn are ameliorated, primarily as a result of reduced gastric acid production. However, gastritis must be treated with caution. The pancreas also reduces its digestive activities and insulin production. In addition, cell receptors develop increased sensitivity for insulin. This is particularly beneficial to diabetics. Fasting normalizes the intestinal flora, which improves immunity. Decreased chronic fatigue and receding inflammatory complaints may result.

Allergies and Inflammatory Disorders

When a person stops ingesting food, he/she also stops ingesting foreign substances that usually enter the body with the food. This relieves the immune system, especially the intestinal immune system as this system is in charge of dealing with these foreign substances. Inflammatory conditions and allergies improve as a result. Nutrition today contains many allergens owing to the variety of foods and the amount of industrial additives. Did you know that in industrialized countries people come in contact with approximately 150 food allergens per day, which increases the probability of developing allergies? The contact with allergens is limited to approximately 10 to 12 in people who live in an undisturbed natural environment and 4 to 10 during therapeutic fasting.

KNOWLEDGE

Fasting—A Break for the Gastrointestinal Tract and the Immune System

- The digestive juices (gastric acid, bile, pancreatic and intestinal secretions) and the wave-like movement of the intestines (peristalsis) are reduced to a minimum.
- The intestinal flora are restored as pathological bacteria cannot feed on anything (substrate).
- The intestinal mucous membrane recedes temporarily.
- The absorption of nutritional antigens and allergens as well as inflammatory substances is suspended.

The beneficial effects of therapeutic fasting that lead to the conclusion that fasting is also beneficial in the case of arteriosclerosis include receding cardiac disorders and mitigation of complaints in the lower extremities, as well as decreasing the risk factors for cardiovascular disorders, including abdominal adiposity, hypertension, hyperlipidemia, diabetes

transported through the walls of the digestive tract and reach all cells, which they supply with energy and building blocks. This process is conducted with the aid of stomach, liver, and pancreatic secretions. The organs of digestion are often overworked due to excessive eating. If the fasting period is stress-free, they can take a break and restore themselves. Gastritis and

My Allergy Story

Every spring I suffer from a seasonal pollen allergy. I am especially bothered by birch pollen, but other spring bloomers trouble me as well.

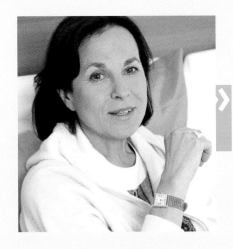

This allergy first appeared 20 years ago, after my second pregnancy. My immune system was weakened by lack of sleep, job stress, and child care, all of which I was very passionate about. Suddenly, in adulthood, I developed symptoms including burning eyes and nasal congestion, which were so severe that I had to stay in bed feeling truly sick. I was barely able to breathe at night. The arsenal of allergy and asthma medication on the market today was not yet available then. What was I to do? Once again, it was fasting and the targeted reduction of food diversity before and after the fast that helped me. While fasting, I can go for walks during birch blossom time without experiencing any symptoms. Of course I feel my eyes reacting when I rub them, but there is

> Fasting, as well as food reduction and the avoidance of cross-allergens, reduces the discomforts of a pollen allergy.

no comparison to the severe symptoms I used to suffer from. I cannot heal the allergy but I can reduce the symptoms.

Reducing the Allergen Load
The immune system, especially the intestinal immune system, is relieved by the reduced allergen load while fasting. The limitation of foods ingested before and after the fast pursues the same goal. Only 10 to 12 different foods should be eaten, avoiding the so-called cross-allergens. In cross-allergies, sensitization to certain inhaled allergens, for example, birch pollen, is followed by an allergic response to botanically related foods, for example, apples.

Avoiding Cross-allergens
I try to schedule my fast during the main birch blossom season. I start off with a diet that contains only 10 different foods. From this reduced selection of foods I exclude all cross-allergens pertaining to me, including hazelnuts, stone fruits, apples (during the rest of the year I can eat some cultivars, but not during allergy season), alcohol, wheat flour, and all products containing gluten. I eat hardly any dairy products with the exception of some curd cheese.

Fasting during the Allergy Season
I recommend fasting during the allergy season and reducing the numbers of foods to be consumed before and after, if you are allergic to pollen and experience seasonal symptoms like I do. Foods have to be chosen depending on your allergens. The most frequent cross-reaction is the one that I experience, the birch-nut-stone-fruits syndrome. We recommend categorically avoiding alcohol, dairy products, and grain products containing gluten during this allergy season. After the allergy season has passed, these foods may be reintroduced.

31

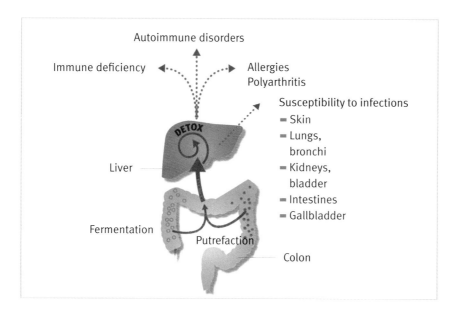

Autoimmune disorders

Immune deficiency

Allergies
Polyarthritis

Susceptibility to infections
- Skin
- Lungs, bronchi
- Kidneys, bladder
- Intestines
- Gallbladder

DETOX

Liver

Fermentation

Putrefaction

Colon

◀ The »toxic colon,« a naturopathic working hypothesis regarding the development of diseases.

Nutrition, individual digestive conditions, and eating habits (especially eating when under stress) can promote the development of a »toxic colon.« These processes of fermentation and decomposition recede while fasting, which provides great relief to the liver and the immune system.

Recession of Intestinal Mucous Membrane

It has been observed in animals that during a fast, the thickness of the intestinal walls tends to decrease. In rats, after a few days of fasting, the typical intestinal villi flatten. Only a few hours after the rats had begun to eat again, the villi were rebuilt swiftly. In humans, this phenomenon has also been noted after long periods of a starvation diet. The obvious thought is that the large intestinal surface (approximately 200 to 600 m²) can act as protein storage. Some fasting experts interpret this ability to break down and rebuild the intestinal surface as a great therapeutic potential in terms of healing colitis and other inflammatory diseases of the digestive tract.

In this case, the return to a regular diet must be realized carefully and gradually. It definitely requires medi-

Precursors of fatty acids promoting inflammation, for example, arachidonic acid contained in meat, dairy, and meat products, are also eliminated while fasting. This results in amelioration of inflammatory processes, for example, of joints, which may result in reduced swelling and regaining mobility.

»Toxic Colon«

Bacteria can already be found in the large intestine right after birth. They enter from the environment and are thus foreign to the newborn, yet indispensable for humans. We call them the intestinal flora.

These microorganisms (400 different species) live in harmony within the intestines of their host, as long as

nutritional and digestive processes run smoothly. If, for example, partially digested portions of food enter the large intestine, bacteria of fermentation and decomposition increase excessively and produce toxic substances and gases, which results in flatulence and abdominal discomfort. The toxic colon content can enter the blood via the thin intestinal and vascular membranes, especially if these membranes are permeable. The intestinal immune system and the liver can neutralize the toxic matter unless they become overwhelmed by them. In this case, toxins enter the organs of elimination, where they cause chronic disorders (e.g., bladder infections, recurring infections of the upper respiratory tract, constipation). Toxins can now enter cells and cause various diseases, depending on individual disposition, if the process continues.

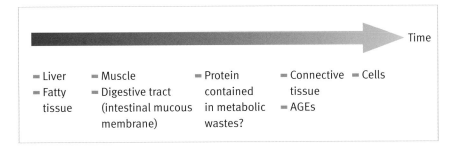

- Liver
- Fatty tissue
- Muscle
- Digestive tract (intestinal mucous membrane)
- Protein contained in metabolic wastes?
- Connective tissue
- AGEs
- Cells

Time

◀ Protein sources during the fast.

cal supervision. In a study by the Norwegian researcher Kjeldsen-Kragh, foods were reintroduced one by one. The foods that produced symptoms were then eliminated from the diet.

Water and Salt Removal

Fasting offers the natural opportunity to eliminate excess salt and water. Abnormal water retention (edema) caused by cardiac or venous insufficiencies, for example, in the lower extremities, may disappear during the first days of a fast. The emptying of the digestive tract, as well as the release of water bonded to glycogen and protein, increase water elimination. These processes can cause plethoric people (people frequently suffering from hypertension, abdominal adiposity, and whose face is reddened) to lose up to 1 L of fluids per day (more than 1 kg per day) during the first week of the fast. They feel liberated. In the further course of fasting, the daily water elimination decreases. The kidneys react to the initial water

removal with the production of aldosterone, a hormone that counteracts sodium elimination. The body now retains the sodium. When returning to a regular diet, salt consumption should be minimal during the first days as the body »craves« it. This means that bread, cheese, and ready-to-use foods should be eaten sparingly as they contain a lot of sodium.

Protein Reduction

The »protein pool« existing in the human body may be compared with a forest. If we need wood, we pick up old branches from the ground and cut down old and damaged trees. When this is done the forest can thrive. It is the same when fasting: the body relies on its own »protein pool« if no proteins are ingested. The body recycles the protein and utilizes it for cellular and structural renewal and gluconeogenesis. During a fast, protein sources include the liver, muscles, intestinal mucous membranes, protein structures of fat and connective

tissues, and possibly intra- or extra-cellular protein metabolic waste.

From a naturopathic point of view, fasting offers the opportunity to metabolize old, pathological, and dispensable protein structures or molecules, and rid cells and connective tissue of their burden.

» Fasting is like surgery without a lancet. It cuts away the superfluous and spares what is healthy.«
Erwin Hof

It is a complicated mechanism that breaks down protein in a body cell. Denaturized or incorrectly folded proteins are selected and folded anew or taken apart to be available for synthesis at other locations. Denaturized and foreign proteins include antigen/antibody-immune complexes, proteins damaged by free radicals, cross-linked proteins as a result of tanning, nonenzymatic AGEs (advanced glycation end products or immune complexes), for example, carcinogen acrylamides contained in potato chips and French fries. It makes sense that they are »self-digested« during a fast. According to the German researcher Lothar Wendt, microcirculation, as well as gas and nutrition exchange between blood and cells, improves after the elimination of pathological protein deposits.

33

Solution to the Mystery on Page 7

No one needs to be afraid of protein utilization; the migratory birds show us how it works. The birds utilize their fat reserves as the primary source of energy, which makes them continuously lose weight. The same effort now requires less muscle mass from the wings and the heart as the bird is lighter.

The conclusion is that very active animals can mobilize, without harm, small amounts of protein from active muscle groups including the heart. Once they reach their destination, they eat and rebuild fat tissue as well as muscle mass until they regain their initial weight. I would like to take the liberty of speculating on the following: protein located in the muscles and other tissues bonds with a significant amount of water. Consequently, even small amounts of protein release water when they are metabolized during a fast. This way, the bird brings its food and water along for the journey.

Cardiovascular Relief

Switching to internal nutrition and quieting of the gastrointestinal tract causes changes in the cardiovascular system. The diminished amount of fluid in the blood, the tissues, and the abdominal area (where fat tissue diminishes as well), together with the parasympathetic activity, results in the relief of the cardiovascular system. Blood pressure and pulse rate are reduced. The performance of the cardiac muscle increases in the course of a fast especially when combined with the proper exercise program, especially after the second week.

Modification of Blood Coagulation

Fasting brings about a natural decrease of blood coagulation, comparable to some medications (e.g., warfarin). People who take coagulation inhibitors, for example, preventive or after venous thrombosis, should have their dosage adapted by a medical doctor.

Aversion to Smoking

People who undergo some sort of weight-reducing diet often begin to drink more coffee and smoke more cigarettes than they did before dieting. In contrast, with the Buchinger Amplius fasting program it has been noted that patients spontaneously smoke less or quit smoking completely, with astoundingly little effort.

The following statistics document this phenomenon:
- Approximately 50% of smokers quit smoking completely
- More than 45% smoke less
- Less than 5% smoke the same

Indications and Contraindications

» Maria Buchinger worked with her father for many years and also conducted his correspondences. One day she asked him: »What are the disorders fasting can improve or cure?« Otto Buchinger answered: »You will have to find an easier question! Rather ask what it is that fasting cannot cure. This list of disorders is short: tuberculosis, hyperthyroidism, and advanced stages of cancer. In all other cases, especially in chronic disorders, it is worth a try.«

The following list of indications and contraindications was compiled by a group of experts as part of the *Guidelines for Therapeutic Fasting*. The list is based on documented experience and the results of scientific research. The indications are only applicable when fasting under medical supervision.

Fasting—Indications

Preventive fasting

Lowering of risk factors:	▪ Overweight ▪ Increased triglycerides, cholesterol, and uric acid levels ▪ Stress ▪ Diabetes mellitus type II ▪ Hypertension ▪ Smoking

Therapeutic fasting

Cardiovascular diseases:	▪ Coronary heart disease (arteriosclerosis of the coronary vessels) ▪ Cardiac insufficiency ▪ Arterial circulatory disorder ▪ Venous insufficiency (edema, leg ulcer)
Back and joint disorders:	▪ Degenerative: arthrosis, arthritis ▪ Inflammatory: rheumatoid arthritis, ankylosing spondylitis
Disorders of the digestive system:	▪ Functional gastrointestinal disorders ▪ Chronic inflammatory intestinal disorders ▪ Chronic constipation
Chronic liver disorders	
General condition:	▪ Mental and physical exhaustion ▪ Symptoms of depression ▪ Chronic fatigue
Various disorders:	▪ Susceptibility to infections (upper respiratory tract, sinuses, bladder) ▪ Migraine and headache ▪ Allergies (asthma, hay fever), neurodermitis ▪ Male and female fertility disorders ▪ Menopausal disorders ▪ Premenstrual syndrome (PMS) ▪ Fibromyalgia ▪ Glaucoma ▪ Acne

Fasting—Contraindications

Absolute contraindications

▪ Cachexia (severe weight loss)
▪ Anorexia nervosa
▪ Decompensated hyperthyroidism
▪ Advanced impairment of cerebral perfusion
▪ Advanced liver or kidney insufficiency
▪ Pregnancy or nursing

Relative contraindications, conditions presenting a risk. Experienced medical care is mandatory.

▪ Addictions (alcohol, eating disorders, drugs)
▪ Gastric, duodenal ulceration
▪ Advanced coronary heart disease
▪ Retinal detachment
▪ Psychosis
▪ Diabetes mellitus type I
▪ Malignant diseases (cancer)

Psychological Effects of Fasting

Fasting as a holistic method not only works on a physical level but also harmonizes the psyche. Most people who fast regularly look forward to the fast for weeks in advance because they have already experienced the sense of well-being that comes with it. An internist I know takes no stock in fasting. The mere idea of not eating for several hours scares him because he envisions the »depletion« his body must endure. It is all a matter of attitude!

A person with experience in fasting knows that the feeling of hunger subsides and is gone after a few hours. Someone else imagines wandering around like a hungry wolf and being stressed for many days on end. The Minnesota study, dating back to 1956, showed that soldiers who were sent into the desert for 35 days and given half of their usual food portion became aggressive or depressed. The expression »dieting depression« (weight-reduction depression) was coined. By now this interpretation has been corrected. Proper weight reduction programs as well as fasting lift the spirit and self-esteem, provided they are carried out deliberately and under expert care. Many people, especially physicians and dietary experts, who went hungry during war, show a negative response to the word fasting. It is nearly impossible to change their minds. Contrary to this reaction, the younger generation is by far more open to fasting and self-awareness. Physicians specializing in fasting can confirm that during in-patient fasting, the mood improves generally within a few days or even hours. This can include spontaneous feelings of happiness and euphoric conditions. Today, these processes are documented on internationally recognized questionnaires about quality of life.

Survey

In a 40-year study in our clinic, we asked 372 patients, who had fasted more than 10 times each in our clinic: »What experience was particularly positive during your fast?« The answers are listed in quantitative order:
1. Well-being, increased vitality
2. Internal harmony, stabilization
3. Detachment from everyday problems / regenerative break
4. Stress reduction
5. Contemplation
6. Problem-solving

KNOWLEDGE

Attitude is Key

»Deliberate fasting and religious fasting rituals have particular psychological effects,« concludes Gerald Huether, neurobiologist in Göttingen, Germany. His studies with animals, as well as with humans during their stay in a fasting clinic, show that fasting intensifies the effects of the neurotransmitter serotonin. Serotonin is a neurotransmitter known to produce positive mood as a result of continuous harmonization of the entire nervous system. Huether also makes some interesting observations regarding stress hormones (adrenalin, noradrenalin, and cortisol) in association with fasting. After a brief rise in stress hormone levels, the levels drop below the initial value if people fast deliberately. If people are forced to go without food, the levels continuously rise. This documents the importance of attitude.

» Some sort of detachment and relaxation of the tense mental structure is noticeable, including inner harmony and heightened sensitivity. Analytic thinking is initially complicated; intuition is more intense and facilitated.«

Dr. Otto Buchinger, in *The Therapeutic Fasting Cure* (*Das Heilfasten*)

Fasting Does Not Mean Starving

» Deliberate fasting can prompt realizations and awareness regarding one's integrity. In this respect, fasting is a method that, in modern terms, is classified as a »vision quest.« Starvation on the other hand, prompts feelings of fear and frustration. The person experiencing this type of hunger is under pressure, remains stressed, and fears for his/her life. The harmonizing effects of serotonin are masked by restlessness and the search for food. This refers primarily to chronic famine and malnutrition.

There are other situations when people deliberately starve themselves, such as hunger strike and anorexia, and also methods for weight reduction including jaw wiring, gastric balloon, and gastric banding, which is a surgical reduction of the stomach that only allows small amounts of food to be ingested.

You may ask yourself legitimately whether a person should be considered starving after such a surgery or if it is possible to truly affirm the forced abstention and maintain the same attitude as a person fasting. The former possibility can lead to uncontrolled eating and fast weight gain once the gastric banding is removed.

Forced fasting imposed by religious institutions can initiate this sort of starvation instead of revealing the liberating vision of therapeutic fasting. Some fasting people put themselves under so much pressure in terms of weight reduction that there is no chance for some internal space to open. In this respect, they need to be considered »starving« rather than »fasting« and psychotherapeutic measures may be helpful as part of the expert care accompanying their fast.

» Everyone can perform magic and everyone can reach their goals, if he can think, if he can wait, and if he can fast.«

Hermann Hesse, *Siddhartha*

Conversely, a forced situation that suggests starvation may change into deliberate fasting. My cousin, an overweight man with fasting experience, had to have his tonsils removed. After the surgery he suffered from severe difficulties in swallowing and was unable to eat. He was supposed to receive intravenous nutrition, but he strictly objected and began fasting. This expedited healing and weight reduction was a welcome side-benefit.

Generally, humans possess the inner freedom to alter starving into fasting; especially if it is about temporary food deprivation and they are experienced in fasting.

▶ A: Fasting does not mean starving: the proper attitude toward fasting brings about inner growth.

B: Constraint and involuntariness bring about starvation.

A

Internal Growths

Serenity, contemplation, releasing the emotional break, restoration of a sound sensibility, reducing fear, high spirit

Fasting

Deliberation

Methodical medical care

Acceptance of the fast by the social environment

The fasting person is the subject of the process

Dietetics of the soul

Positive attitude

Experiencing one's own body

Escaping the daily routine

Group experience

B

Involuntary

Chronic famine

Destitution, war, poverty, loss

Family and »experts« warn about pseudo-dangers

The starving person is the victim of the process

Lack of spiritual–psychological care

Lack of physical care

Duress, control

Starving

Food obsession, stress, fear, suffering, apathy, depression, deficiency symptoms

How Does the Mind Change?

» It is amazing how fasting spontaneously and physiologically intensifies the harmonizing effects of serotonin on the brain. Nowadays, people usually take psychotropic drugs to achieve the same results. There are a number of stimulating and reviving effects during a fast, such as the holiday feeling and the group experience, soothing massages, detachment from stress factors, and the temporary deliberate separation from partners, friends, and family. Some additional effects, very specific to fasting, will be discussed below. These experiences can guide fasting people back to their existential truth, by helping them to leave their beaten paths.

Feeling the Self-healing Power

It is not uncommon during a fast that joint pain recedes within a short period of time and movement improves; blood pressure normalizes despite the prediction of lifelong medication;

headache, hay fever, or skin disorders disappear. Experiences like that induce high spirits, hope, and confidence in one's own self-healing powers.

It has become a rare occasion that a person has the chance to consciously experience e.g., the ceasing of a headache without medicinal aids. The affected person is astounded by their self-healing potential while fasting.

Breaking Behavior Patterns

Today we typically encounter overworked people who are caught in a vicious cycle of excessive work and food and not enough sleep. Possibly their social network is limited and they neglect their relationships. One morning they wake up and think: »This cannot continue. I must do something!« Fasting offers a chance to break with all behavior patterns, in particular with those that are imbalanced and disease-causing. Away from the structures of everyday life, a new balance can be gained.

More Time

The heavenly feeling of not being pressured by time is the first reward for a fasting person. No time must be spent preparing meals and sitting down to eat. This also eliminates other activities such as grocery shopping and cleaning up after a meal. The person lives on »autopilot« and is supplied from their internal stores as needed without engaging mental activity or will.

》 The famous artist Günther Uecker describes this with the following words: ›When I fast I can spend hours on a meadow watching a blade of grass moving in the wind. While fasting, time is not broken up and shaped by the rhythm of hunger and satiety. I can move from exhaustion to creation.‹«

KNOWLEDGE

The Serotogenic System

Information processing in the brain is an integrative process in which countless stimuli gathered from the sensory organs and other cerebral regions are composed to form an internal impression. The integration process for such variety of information always produces some unrest. Several comprehensive systems settle this unrest to facilitate the harmonization and beneficial processing of different stimuli. One of these systems acts through the release of the neurotransmitter serotonin and is hence called the »serotogenic system.« The brain is flooded rhythmically with small amounts of serotonin, several times per second. The neurotransmitter regulates the stimuli and processing that takes place in various regions of the brain. Once the task is accomplished, the serotonin is returned to the cells by something comparable to little vacuum cleaners. Such vacuum cleaners can be slowed down in their activity, which intensifies the harmonizing effect and turns it into lasting feelings of happiness. This is the effect that fasting exerts on the serotogenic system. The same effect is achieved through medication such as antidepressants, or illegal drugs such as ecstasy. The serotonin release following ecstasy abuse is so enormous, however, that it depletes the brain. Foods containing ample amounts of fat and sugar (e.g., chocolate, potato chips) also increase the serotonin release and make us happy, for a short time only!
(Gerald Huether: »The unconscious manipulation of mood and feelings through food intake«, original in German)

KNOWLEDGE

The Intestines—The Second Brain

Research shows that an important neural structure (the Auerbach plexus / Meissner plexus) continuously »analyzes« the intestinal environment and passes the information on to the cerebral centers. Depending on the conditions, the health of the intestines and their flora (bacterial colonization) as well as decomposition and fermentation processes have an impact on the mood. The origin of this word reveals that melancholics (*melancholia*: Greek for »black bile«), whose gallbladder dysfunction affects the digestive process, tend to be depressed and apathetic. The person with a stocky »pyknic« physique, whose digestive system is well developed, is a rather cheerful type. The interplay between the health of the intestines and mood is well known. The quieting of the gastrointestinal tract and the disappearance of unhealthy intestinal flora that are not fed while fasting is reported to the brain as good news of peace and harmony.

A »space in time« arises. Some fasting people enjoy the quiet and solitude. Others feel the urge to do things that they usually do not find the time for, like cleaning up a room, finishing something that was long due, writing a letter, going to a concert, or spending time on art, dancing, or playing. When time and space are available, one may find access to his/her creativity and a new world of experiences. People who have not drawn a picture since pre-school suddenly take up a brush or they dare to sing or write.

Different Quality of Sleep

During the course of the fast, the need for sleep decreases. Another gain in time! The quality of time at night is different from its quality during the day, therefore, fasting is traditionally associated with being awake. The special qualities of feeling and thinking during the night can be revealed. In association with dreams, these nocturnal experiences can lead to revelations or even small »enlightenments.« Indifference to being awake at night is feasible because the next day does not pose any demands; one can sleep in or rest during the midday break.

»Dematerialization«

In place of the digestion of material foods, the body switches to a sort of virtual nutrition while fasting. The abdominal space calms down. In metaphorical terms, this could be called a form of »dematerialization.« The fasting person switches into a metabolic state that represents the very antithesis of consumption.

Some people experience the sensation of being at one with cosmic forces, for example while going for a morning walk or for a swim in the lake. The fasting person does not experience physical hunger—he or she is ready for the dietetics of the soul. This person is ready to open to a world of refined perception. Christianne Méroz speaks of the everyday mysticism that becomes accessible through marveling, curiosity, awareness, dreaming, and ultimately bliss. Known words have new meaning to fasting people.

Heightened Senses

Indeed, many fasting people report an elevated sensibility toward sensory perceptions. »As if my eyes see the richness of colors and shapes in a new light.« »I have never perceived odors as intensely as during my fast.«

» Abstention does not take. Abstention gives. It gives the inexhaustible power of simplicity.«

Martin Heidegger

One thing is for certain: when beginning to eat again after the fast, simple foods like an apple or potato soup

▶ A feeling of ease and freedom may arise during the fast.

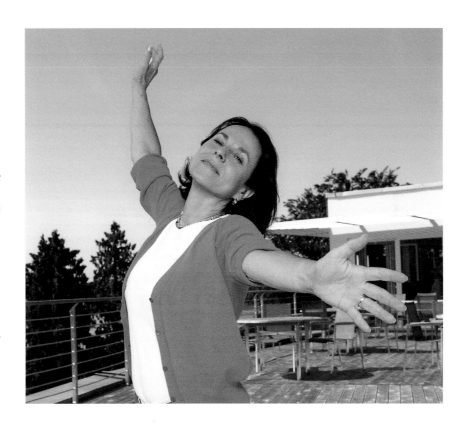

taste absolutely delicious. One of the great secrets of fasting is that there is no loss of pleasure.

You may ask: »Where is the pleasure in not eating?« Fasting turns out to be a space of more subtle pleasures; the lesser the consumption, the greater is the ability to enjoy.

Letting Go

Giving up the control over eating habits in order to switch the energy supply onto autopilot is part of learning the art of letting go. The rhythm of fasting is slower but more intense. The fasting person depends on fat, which is in charge of long-term but submaximal performance.

Sugar (glucose), the accelerator, has to be used sparingly. The sphere of »slow food« is entered. Letting go is the theme of all forms of meditation, therefore, fasting can be considered a type of body meditation. In addition, every fast is a symbolic exercise of mirthful dying. A former physician specializing in fasting is of the opinion, like the Indians, that when the time of dying has arrived it is best to begin fasting.

KNOWLEDGE

Eating Out of Frustration—Consciously Experienced

An American music lover became seriously concerned during his first fast because listening to one of his favorite Bach pieces brought on an unprecedented feeling of happiness. We calmed him and recommended he simply dedicate himself to this feeling. A key experience followed: he received a phone call from his company in New York during one of his musical »trances.« Even though there was no bad news, he experienced a desire to eat that he had not had for days. Being torn out of his state of bliss, he reacted with the craving for food. Mental frustrations are often blocked out with food.

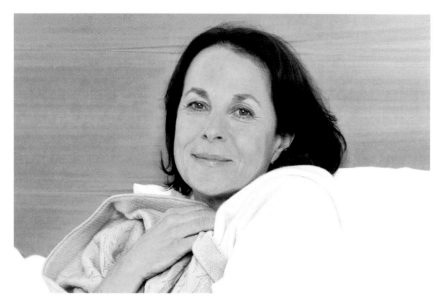

▲ Listen to your »inner child«: what does it need right now? Security, being mothered, or physical closeness?

Dr. Otto Buchinger himself died when he was 89 years old, surrounded by a few close family members. He knew that it was time to »go home« as he put it. His peaceful death will always be remembered by his family. Did his long-time fasting experience help him?

The »Inner Child«

Therapeutically guided fasting offers the opportunity to receive attention and be »in touch« with body and soul. It also allows feeling and experiencing the world like a child. In order to admit this »therapeutic regression,« the fasting person must feel safe and cared for. Many natural treatments, including wraps, massages, heat and moisture applications, as well as colon cleansing imply that we grant therapists access to our privacy. Fasting people may experience periods of weakness and should therefore rest at midday. This state is quite conducive to accepting being mothered and touched. Once the regression into childhood has been permitted, emotions are freed and tears often may flow freely. We get the chance to acknowledge our unfulfilled needs and develop adequate coping strategies.

»Returning to the Womb«

In the womb, the fetus receives nourishment directly from the maternal blood through the placenta. Its digestive tract is still at rest and yet the fetus grows and flourishes. As soon as the baby is born it depends on its own digestive tract for its nutrition. As an adult, fasting is a symbolic return to the womb. The fasting person lives off stored food, primarily fat, which is delivered directly into his/her blood and, just like with the fetus, the digestive tract is at rest. It is suggested that one compares birth with breaking a fast, which explains the title of a fasting guidebook: *Reborn through Fasting*. The fasting person is surrounded by a number of protective layers, like in the womb, including the fasting retreat, the fasting community, the institution with its team of therapists, and, in case of religious fasting, the religious community. Symbolically, fasting regularly can mean to be continuously reborn.

New Horizons

An important psychological momentum during a fast is when a person realizes that he/she feels neither weak nor hungry but vital and content. »If I have the unimagined ability to do this, I can also push other limits.«

Mental Contraindications

» How is your mental health? Are your basic needs (see box) met? Do you have healthy strategies at hand to cope with fear, frustration, and emotional shortcomings? Do you consider yourself psychologically healthy and stable? Psychologically stable people can fast without concerns. Nevertheless, fasting crises may occur. The next section talks about how to deal with them. You should contact a physician with fasting experience or a psychologist if you know or believe that you are emotionally out of balance. Their expertise can help you to clarify whether fasting is the right thing to do at the moment, for example, if you are:

- emotionally unstable;
- suffering from an eating disorder, including anorexia, bulimia, or binge eating;
- addicted to alcohol or drugs;
- taking psychotropic or other drugs related to mental disorders.

If the fasting expert considers it advisable for you to fast, you should plan on in-patient fasting in a clinic. This is the only approach that provides medical and psychotherapeutic support in a timely manner if needed. People with fasting experience consciously utilize the fast to work through a life crisis or critical decision, to mourn a lost person, or process other life crises. I recommend doing so in the shelter of a fasting clinic just the same.

What to do During a Fasting Crisis?

» In the course of a fast, various »traps« and challenges may present themselves. I will now outline how you can use these situations as a chance for personal growth and development. Below I will use the term »syndrome« when referring to a common pattern. I use this term simply because it is handy and not to be derogatory or to classify something as being pathological.

Packing-the-bags Syndrome

»Why am I doing this to myself?« That is what some people may think at the beginning of the fast. Everything seems so arduous. The physical adaptation from outer to inner nutrition may present discomfort. One feels restless and uncomfortable. This is a fertile soil for doubts. Do not fight them but stay with the feelings inside of you. Ask yourself: why do I feel so uncomfortable? What can I do about it? Accept help. After a little while you will be glad not to have succumbed to the temptation to pack your bags and leave, in other words not to have quit fasting. Maybe it comforts you to know that the packing-the-bags syndrome is a very common phenomenon. Experience teaches us to meet these moments of doubt with a smile.

Loss-of-the-mental-crutch Syndrome

The fasting person waives smoking, alcohol, maybe recreational drugs, or gambling, as well as activities that, when engaged in excessively, take on a compensative function, for example, work, social activities, and even sex. That means that during the fast a person gives up some crutches that make everyday life easier. The compensation for this is: soul food! Soul food includes art, creativity, humor, nature, relationships, and spirituality. Take a look at pages 14–17. What appeals to you? What do you need right now?

Fat and sweet foods may be such a crutch for overweight people, an indulgence that may be employed as a coping strategy for fears and shortcomings. The emotions can become imbalanced if this crutch is unavailable during a fast. A search for new coping strategies is required. In this situation, it is helpful to communicate with others, participate in psychotherapy, and to keep a diary.

Catharsis

Negative emotions that have been denied and calamities that have not been processed properly may surface into consciousness while fasting. Mental crises during a fast appear as sudden depression, bursting into tears, or in the form of physical symptoms, including food cravings or discomfort. It is the responsibility of the specialists accompanying the fast (physician, psychologist, minister) to assess whether this is primarily a physical disorder or a so-called healing crisis. The healing crisis offers the opportunity to experience denied emotions in a safe environment and to work out resolution strategies via emphatic conversations.

Record-setting Syndrome

Some people want to set fasting records. A word of caution: there is an opportunity to be injudicious and exceed the appropriate fasting period. See the next chapter for advice about how long to fast.

FROM MY EXPERIENCES

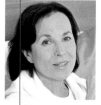

It Makes it Easier to Love My Body

While I am fasting I completely calm down within a few days. I can call on my inner calm and serenity. Order and punctuality come about without effort, different from everyday life. I directly perceive the effects that my emotions have on my body. I cry more easily and fear seems almost palpable in my stomach, throat, and heart. It feels as if there is no distance between my perceptions and myself. The tendency to »pathologically« criticize, judge, and label myself and my surroundings recedes. I feel with my five senses instead: scents in nature (unfortunately including car exhaust), landscapes through my window or facial expressions of people around me, subtle sounds and inner voices, impressions on the skin, the hand of the massage therapist, the water of the lake while swimming between mountains and meadows, and the sun warming my sometimes shivering body. It makes it easier to love my body and to be grateful for the many sensations that it awards me.
I would like to remain this conscious, even when the fast is over.

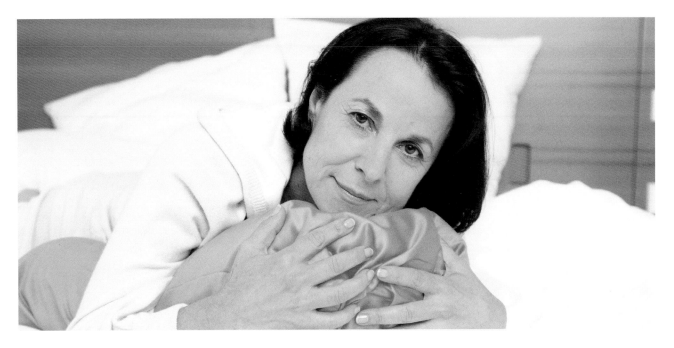

Not-wanting-to-come-down Syndrome

Especially toward the end of a fast, the desire may arise to remain within the serotogenic harmony of fasting. In this case, accept to »fast to the fasting experience«: just accept the next step: the break of the fast.

Internal Obstacles

Internal obstacles arise when fears (often unconscious ones) are not acknowledged. The following behavior patterns and symptoms may be indicators for such obstacles:

- Excessive activities
- Excessive treatments
- Fantasies about food, talking about food
- Excessive focus on weight reduction
- Physical symptoms
- Hypochondria, fear
- Feeling hungry
- Sleep disorders
- Constant fatigue

How can these obstacles be reduced?
- Have a specialized physician examine the symptoms.
- Try things that make you feel good (exercising, sleeping, bathing, writing, singing, etc.).

- Talk to a specialized psychotherapist, a fasting counselor, or your minister.

45

Experiences: When and Why Do We Fast?

Fasting can be helpful in many situations and life circumstances. It brings amelioration and even healing to many physical ailments and diseases.

With very few exceptions, I respond to every disorder with fasting. When my stomach or my intestines are upset I fast until my hunger returns. I also fast when rheumatic discomfort arises and live through my allergy season with minimal discomfort thanks to fasting (see p. 31). I have fasted through all life crises. My existence is shaped by fasting. No matter what happens, my first response is usually fasting (varying from some hours to some days).

Every person is different and responds differently. Below, other people with fasting experience will tell you their story, giving you a more comprehensive impression. Let us ask my husband, Raimund Wilhelmi, when and why he fasts.

Raimund Wilhelmi about the »Physical Tummy«

» I am part of my own target group: I love good food. I do not move enough and am under business stress. I am politically involved: after the official meeting, the true discussions begin, wine flows, and Italian food is eaten until late at night. This leaves its mark around the waist. I counteract that through fasting, which I do at least once a year for 3 to 4 weeks. I lose an average of 10 kg. I schedule this long fasting period for the beginning of the year. Sometimes I fast again for 1 week in autumn. During these fasts my liver counts, cholesterol, blood pressure, and weight adjust. Aside from these positive physical effects, fasting obtains increasing significance in my life as a time for self-reflection.

I think about my path in life and have the time to reflect on certain themes

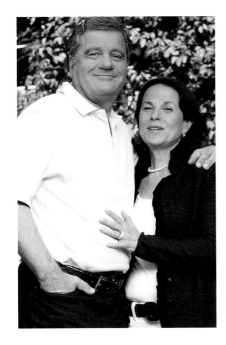

◀ The director of the clinic also fasts regularly.

down there with phones ringing and dogs barking. Now, just like any other guest I move into one of the rooms in our clinic and meet other patients and let myself be treated by our staff. It would not work like that in my own house.

But none of that has turned me into an ascetic. Maybe one day the nature of my grandfather, Dr. Otto Buchinger, will get the upper hand within me. But in all honesty, he did not have the nature of an ascetic either. One of his reasons for fasting was at times that he had ›indulged‹ in eating, not in alcohol or meats—he was vegetarian— but in pastries and cream.«

of my life. I reflect on spiritual issues, the future, and my surroundings. It has turned into a very profound process. I always look forward to it and feel pretty uplifted afterward. I wish to be able to fast for 40 days one time. So far, 20 actual fasting days have been the longest fasting period for me.

Another positive side-effect is that I know our institution from the perspective of our guests. I always fast in our clinic in Überlingen, on Lake Constance.

I used to go to my mother in Marbella to fast, but I was unable to wind

Günter Jena, Church Music Director, Well-known Musician and Bach Specialist, about the »Mental Tummy«

» At 65, I looked back at a life that had included a lot of sitting and unhealthy late-night eating (after rehearsals and concerts), which was part of my profession. I still wanted to look forward to a healthy and interesting life. At that point I fasted at the Buchinger Clinic for the first time.

I learned that a cultural program was part of the everyday clinic routine— true to the motto of its founder Otto Buchinger: ›During the fast the body thrives, but the soul starves. The soul needs food, spiritual food.‹ I gave my first lecture at the clinic. This has turned into a bond that has lasted since 2001 and has regularly brought me back to the clinic to give lectures almost once a month within the last few years. I fast in the clinic once a

year, enjoying the medical care and consultation as well as the variety of offers, including swimming, gymnastics, hiking, and last but not least some miraculous therapies like the breathing therapy.

I see some considerable parallels with making music: not only does our body develop a bit of a tummy, our soul is also ballasted with old habits and debilitating obsessions that are carried around like on a vendor's tray. We have experienced a person or a situation in a certain way and expect that this experience will always repeat itself in the same way. We do not consider that life runs like a river and people also do change. Our physical tummy is not only esthetically unpleasing, but it also threatens our health with its toxic fats. Our mental tummy not only turns us into bores and know-it-alls, but it threatens our soul, because movement and change are part of our physical health as well as of our mental health.

Music and fasting create space for something new; new emotions, and new insights. The physical tummy is fought during a fast. Music can reduce or even eliminate the mental tummy that lures us into the danger of having a one-track mind, because music broadens our emotional perceptiveness, intensifies our emotions, and confronts us with emotions that linger in the distance.

Medicine and fasting are only effective when they are taken or repeated regularly. Music must be listened to over and over to be effective. The best would be to do both regularly: listen to music and fast. The clinic invites you to do so. On that note, I wish the clinic and its guests much success in the future.«

Karl Duschek, Graphic Designer and Logo Specialist (Stankowski + Duschek, Stuttgart)— From Modest to the Finest Esthetics

» ›Why don't you join me?‹, the renowned gallery owner Walter Storms from Munich said to me in the summer of 1991. All right, then. This turned into my first visit to the Buchinger Clinic in the August of 1991. Fasting or organic, vegetarian low-calorie food, I did not really care either way. I was housed at one end of the park villa, which is the most modest place on the premises. I tried everything back then; massages, hay wraps, therapeutic exercises, hikes, and so on.

Finally I experienced the actual effects of fasting that were later confirmed by others, for example Günther Uecker. The urge to do something, to be active and to change something about this world becomes overwhelming. I wrote a book, my most successful book so far. *Visual Communication* has become a standard reference and required reading for all students and faculty of graphic design. At the time there was one problem though: nurse Renate had caught me smoking behind the house. ›I will report this to the clinic management,‹ the dutiful employee said. That stirred me the entire time.

I have returned to Überlingen almost every year and become sort of an insider with my own agenda: resting, bicycling, swimming, and nothing else. Getting older and heavier I even started to care for fasting itself. But the primary reason for my stays at Buchinger is the decelerated life in »nothingness.« I love »emptiness.« Despite grave health problems, I ignore the finger-wagging of doctors. The Buchinger world has become my world; the lake, the environment, and the strict basic concept are the best for me. The »big guys« of industry, who have me work as a design artist for them, love to hear my stories about Buchinger, but I guess they could not bring themselves to simply come here and do it.

I designed an anniversary logo for the year 2000. I truly enjoyed doing this work, being familiar with the nature of the clinic. Part of it was a coherent visual conception. I am very pleased to see that this logo has been so positively received and that today it represents »Buchinger.« The harmonious colors and typography support the design of the logo.

Recently I was asked to apply my experience in the art sector to the new construction of the Villa Bellevue. Speaking of art, I must say that Raimund and Françoise Wilhelmi possess fundamental knowledge in this respect, for example being members of the »Friends of the Busch-Reisinger Museum.« Hence, a convincing concept including the functional aspect was in demand. I furnished this great new construction of the Villa Bellevue with art and design, including room numbers, installations in the halls, and original paintings and photo collages in the guest rooms. I was guided by the idea of ease and its visual elements. The color accents are meant to be conducive to their environment. Nothing is meant to be perceived as disruptive. Art and supportive design must feel natural and timeless. This is truly an environment of pure esthetics. I was a guest in the Villa Bellevue recently. What a beautiful building it is; functional and esthetically very pleasing. It is the complete opposite of the modest Park Villa that I stayed at 18 years ago. I since have put on some years and some kilos, but my attitude toward Buchinger has remained unchanged. Losing weight does not matter to me; I enjoy immersing myself in the world of spiritual balance and rest.«

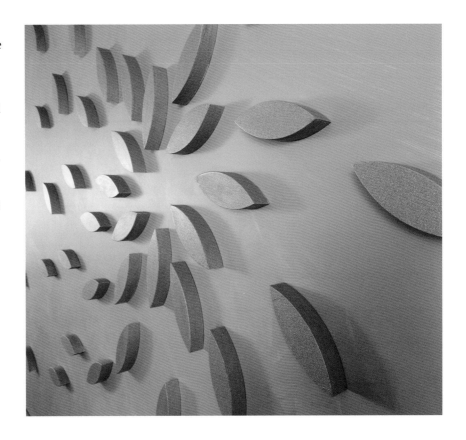

Marie-Jo Lafontaine, Belgian Photo and Video Artist: »I Love Fasting«

» I love fasting because:
- body and soul return to their harmonious state, away from the everyday turmoil;
- it brings more awareness about life, conflicts lose their significance;
- my body is awake and whispers subtle messages;
- my body is in line with feelings regarding the inner and outer world;
- I feel vibrant energy inside of me, I immerse myself in nature;
- minor ailments disappear and so does my migraine;
- food suddenly means something to me;
- it guides my spirit to bright levels of consciousness and opens new spaces.

Fasting is more than a well, it's the source.«

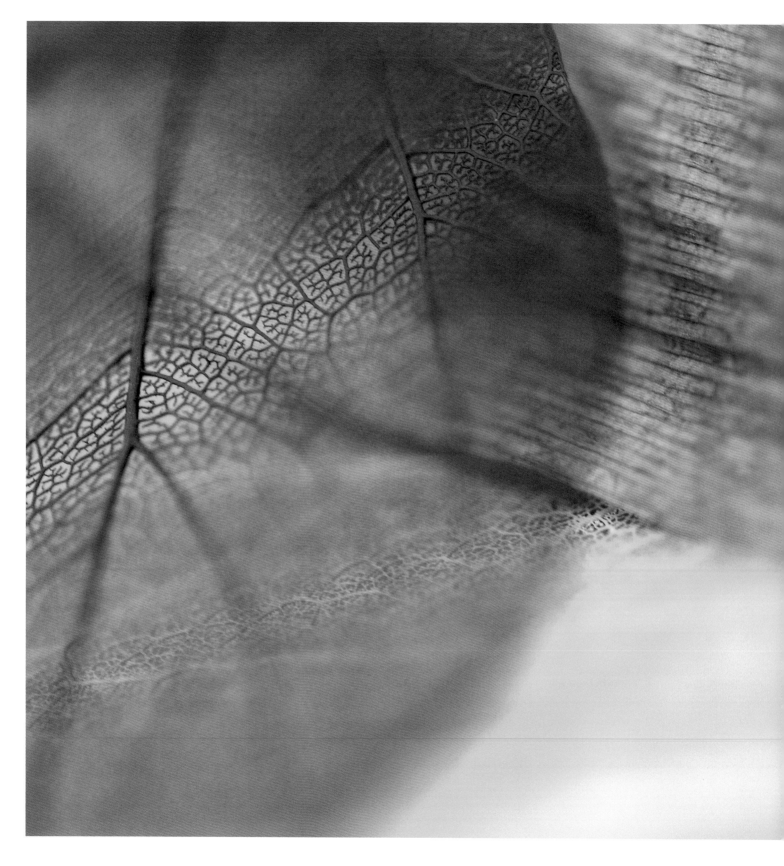

Your Fasting Program

I will now introduce to you in detail all elements of The Buchinger Amplius therapeutic fasting. You will get the essential instructions, learn about helpful exercises, and get numerous pointers for your fasting program. On pages 98 to 99 you will find a table that gives you the outline for a 10-day fast.

Planning Your Individual Fast

It is recommended that you follow a reliable method when you plan your first fast, for example, the Buchinger Amplius fasting program introduced to you in this book. When you repeat fasting, you can increasingly follow your own instincts.

I recommend that for your first fast you consult with an experienced fasting expert, even if you feel physically and mentally healthy and stable. A physician specializing in fasting or a well-educated fasting counselor would serve this purpose. When you fast repeatedly, you will learn to listen to your body and sense what is good for you and which are the best conditions for your fasts.

The Buchinger Amplius fasting program is a three-dimensional »healing fast« (see pp. 10 to 13). Its method rests on seven pillars and was intended to be carried out in a medical center by Dr. Otto Buchinger.

▶ The fast is divided into four phases, which are outlined in this figure.

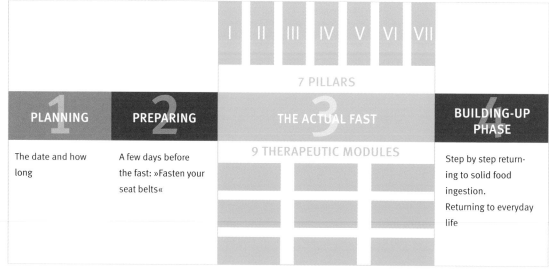

		I II III IV V VI VII	
		7 PILLARS	
1 PLANNING	**2** PREPARING	**3** THE ACTUAL FAST	**4** BUILDING-UP PHASE
		9 THERAPEUTIC MODULES	
The date and how long	A few days before the fast: »Fasten your seat belts«		Step by step returning to solid food ingestion. Returning to everyday life

In the fasting clinics in Überlingen/ Lake Constance, Germany and Marbella, Spain the method is called the Buchinger Amplius fasting method with its nine therapeutic modules.

In the 1980s many fasting variations developed. There were the experience-type and the adult education–type fasts called »fasting for the healthy,« »fasting and hiking,« or »fasting in the monastery.« They can only offer part of the Buchinger Amplius fasting program because these fasts do not have a therapeutic intent. A fasting counselor training was initiated, originally with the idea of supporting the physician. Today, short fasting groups for healthy people are offered by fasting counselors on their own.

How and Where?

I recommend that you consult with an experienced physician whenever you fast. The physician can stay on the sidelines if you are healthy. In this instance, a well-trained fasting counselor can supervise you. The fasting experience is more profound when you manage to remove yourself from everyday life. Should you decide to fast at home, adhering to steady daily routines and rituals helps to detach you from everyday life.

Advantages and disadvantages of different settings

How and where?	Advantages	Disadvantages
Under medical-therapeutic care, possibly with a fasting counselor		
• In a clinic—away from everyday life • With an experienced physician, as part of everyday life or during vacation time	• Physicians and therapists accompany the fast especially in case of physical and mood disorders • Great safety	• Costly (but sensible investment) • Few clinics and doctors' offices offer this care
Under the care of a well-trained fasting counselor and physician on the sidelines		
• In a hotel or monastery, away from everyday life • At home as part of everyday life or during vacation time	• Lower cost • Many attractive offers • Spiritual guidance in a monastery	• Only appropriate for physically and mentally healthy people, who do not take any medications • Fasting only for healthy people • Great differences in the quality of the offers
By oneself without counseling or guidance		
• At home as part of everyday life or during vacation time I only recommend this variation for people with plenty of experience in fasting, who are disciplined in regard to fasting and building up to a regular diet	• Can be started whenever it seems necessary • Low cost	• No safety

When?

» In areas where the religious community celebrates fasting rituals everyone is familiar with the annual fasting season. The community is prepared for this season through prayers and rites.

If you plan the fast yourself, it is advisable to schedule it quite a bit ahead of time. That way you can integrate this time in your plans for the year and attune yourself. Timely planning allows for a harmonious metabolic adaptation of your body to the fast, just like the thought of a meal

initiates the first digestive processes. You can opt for a liturgical period, for example, Lent before Easter, during Ramadan, or around Yom Kippur. You can also schedule a fasting period according to the seasons. For people who like to retreat, autumn or winter may be a good time; others who like to associate a feeling of vacation with their fast may prefer spring or summer. The warm time of the year or a warm climate is certainly preferred by people who feel cold easily. A person with low blood pressure may want to stay in the mountains.

It is important to avoid times when urgent family or business affairs must be tended to.

Fasting Once a Year

When you fast for the first time, you are particularly observant. You watch your body, the new metabolic activities, and new experiences. When you fast for the second time, everything is much more familiar. The more often you fast the more the mental–spiritual dimensions open up to you. Every fast is a new adventure with new experiences. The annual fasting experiences are like milestones in

Christian, Jewish, and Islamic calendar, including Easter, Yom Kippur, and Ramadan

Christian calendar Lent: from Ash Wednesday until Easter		Jewish calendar Yom Kippur		Islamic calendar Ramadan	
Year		Year		Year	
2012	February 21–April 8	5773	September 26	1433	July 21–August 19
2013	February 13–March 31	5774	September 14	1434	July 10–August 9
2014	March 5–April 20	5775	October 4	1435	June 29–July 29
2015	February 18–April 5	5776	September 23	1436	June 18–July 17
2016	February 9–March 27	5777	October 12	1437	June 7–July 7
2017	March 1–April 16	5778	September 30	1438	May 27–June 26
2018	February 14–April 1	5779	September 19	1439	May 16–June 14

one's life or like the »vertebral bodies« of the spine. Every fast can be considered contemplation for taking stock, cleansing the body, setting a new course, and discovering new perspectives.

Spontaneous Decision

In addition to long-term fasting plans, a fast can be decided upon on short notice, for example when there are important decisions to make (do I get married, do I change my residence, do I change my work place?), when mourning and when working through the loss of a loved one. In the case of health disorders or diseases, fasting can help to prevent heavy treatments. People with fasting experience fast spontaneously when noticing the first signs of the flu, or indigestion, weight gain, and joint disorders. Without the necessary fasting experience, medical care should be available. Learn how to fast while you are healthy, because it will give you a good chance to remain healthy and, should you get ill, you are already experienced and can react promptly.

Work or Vacation?

Generally, the fasting rule is along the lines of: »Take the liberty to do what you feel like doing.« We have had guests in our clinic who wrote a book

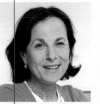

FROM MY EXPERIENCES

Scheduling the Fasting Period

My own experience can serve as an example for scheduling the fast. For the past 30 years, I have fasted in a group annually for 2 weeks at the same location. At the end of each fast, the next fast is scheduled. I write the dates in my empty planner for the next year, including arrival day, transition day, and the days building up to a regular diet. I also make a note about stress prevention for the week prior and after the fasting period. This allows me to prepare myself for the fast and the return to everyday life. In addition to the fasting period, I block out vacation time and schedule all obligations for the remaining time.

or a movie script and others who brought 20 kg of files and took them back without having touched them. If you can afford it, fast without the pressure of having to work!

If you fast at home, take care of pending tasks in the days prior to the fast and make sure that during the fast you have at least 3 hours a day without any obligations.

How Long?

The ideal length of therapeutic fasting (the »Buchinger Amplius classic«) is between 2 and 3 weeks, in a fasting center with personal care by your physician. Individual constitution, health condition and vitality during the fast determine its length. Shorter fasting periods may be advantageous, especially in underweight individuals. Single fasting or detox days can achieve a corrective change in the body. If indicated, longer fasting periods (up to 6 weeks and even longer) may be appropriate. For a therapeutic

fast a minimum of 10 days is recommended. This includes 1 transition day, 5 days fasting, 1 day breaking the fast, and 3 days building-up to a regular diet. In the table on pages 98 to 99, you can find a proposal on how to structure these 10 days.

You may want to try the »fasting week for the healthy,« including 1 transition day (also considered the arrival day), 5 days fasting, and 2 to 4 days building up to a regular diet. This is sometimes done without medical support.

What Do I Need?

Away from everyday life or at home: what do I need? One of the joys of fasting is that one gets along with very few things. Therefore, if you fast away from home, do not overload your luggage. Pack only the important things that you must bring with you, including the following:

- Warm clothes (sweater, socks, scarf, hat, gloves)
- Hiking clothes and boots
- Rain gear
- Bathing suit

- Comfortable clothing (sweat suit, robe)
- Hot-water bottle and a small thin cloth (also provided in the clinic)
- Elegant clothes in case you feel like dressing up
- Body brush or massage glove, tongue scraper, nasal douche, colonic irrigation kit, Vaseline
- Body lotion or oil (organic grade)
- Diary
- Books that you have been meaning to read
- Your favorite music

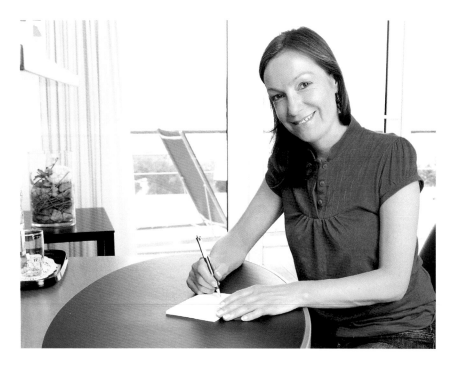

Shopping List

If you are taking care of your »fasting food« yourself, you should buy the following (enough for 5 to 7 fasting days):

- Ca. 3 kg vegetables for the vegetable broth (250 mL daily, see recipe p. 115)
- Organic fruit or vegetable juices (two 1 L bottles or smaller bottles that allow a greater variety), or fresh fruit for juicing 1.5 L
- 1.5 kg fruit or 150 g whole grain rice for the transition days (see recipes pp. 110 to 114)
- Various fresh organic herbal teas, for example, chamomile, linden, peppermint, verbena, or apple tea
- Five organic lemons
- 10 to 15 L mineral water (little or no carbonation)
- 40 g Glauber's salt, available in pharmacies without prescription (dosage see p. 72)
- Some wheat bran in case of colonic sluggishness
- Optional: five low-fat yoghurts and a small bottle of flax seed oil (100 mL); eat one yoghurt a day with 1 teaspoon of flax seed oil added and stirred thoroughly

You can do the shopping for the building-up phase foods on your last day of the fast. Recipes for the building-up phase can be found on pages 116 to 124.

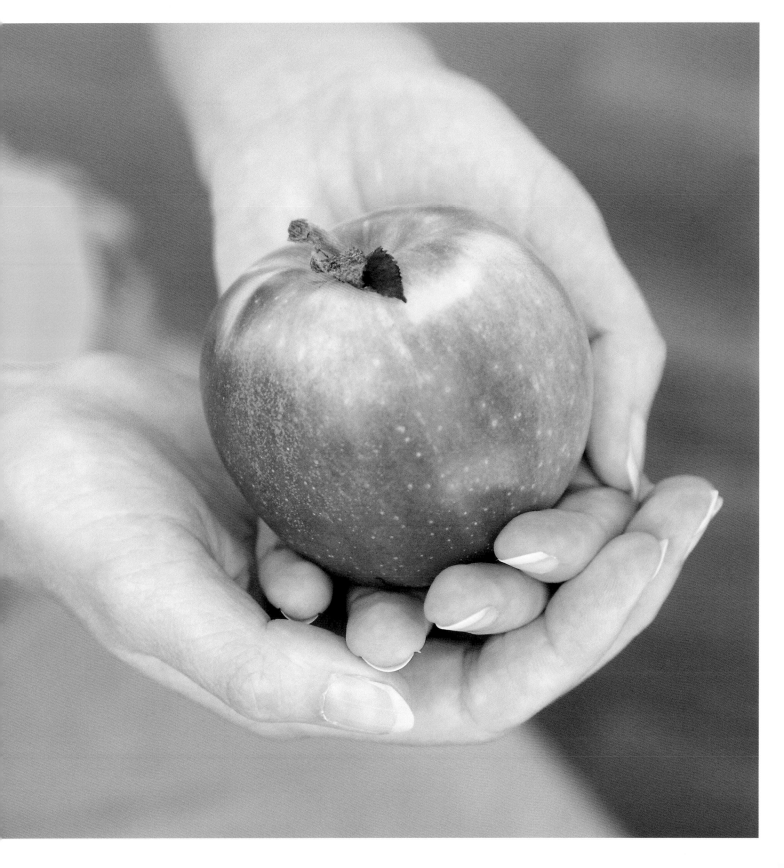

The Seven Pillars of Fasting

No matter which variation of fasting you choose for yourself, the seven pillars apply to each variation from day 1. I will introduce the pillars individually on the following pages.

The more comprehensive the care you receive during the fast, the easier it is to fully realize all seven areas. In regard to adjuvant therapies, people who choose to fast at home must, for example, go on hikes on their own; the ones who choose to stay at a hotel must make appointments for massages and such ahead of time and find out about hiking trails, work-out opportunities and so forth, which requires some organization.

Fasting and Constitution

Before taking a look at the seven pillars you should reflect upon your constitution. Are you exhausted, tired, and pallid with cold extremities and low blood pressure (below 110 mmHg systolic) but without the tendency to be overweight? In this case you probably belong to the »low-vitality-level« category and should treat yourself with great care:

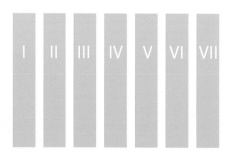

7 PILLARS

1. Serenity, quietness, and relaxation
2. Movement
3. Boosting elimination (»detox«)
4. Adjuvant therapies
5. Care
6. Fasting beverages
7. Soul food

58

- Slow transition into and out of the fasting period, for example, 2 to 3 transition days instead of only 1 day
- Absolutely no stress and no rush
- Warm beverages (you can also drink warm water)
- Warm rooms, warm clothes
- Invigorating treatments (dry brushing, frequent physical activities of medium intensity, warm foot and hand soaks)
- Careful slow return to a regular diet (not too many raw foods)

Contrary to the »low-vitality-level« type, the »plethoric« type displays the following characteristics: heat, reddened face, hypertension, and frequently overweight with abdominal adiposity. The plethoric type usually fasts without difficulties and feels increasing well-being day by day. They do not feel hungry and can handle some physical strain (provided that the cardiovascular system does not suffer any disorder).

Serenity, Quietness, and Relaxation

Take your time. Explore the borderline to boredom and a new space of time will open up, showing you myriads of things and correlations that usually pass unheeded.

Allow yourself to enjoy serenity during the fast. Avoid all stressors and let the rush of everyday life fade. After the adaptation phase, the autonomic nervous system takes command and the digestive system is at rest. Visit nice places while you are fasting, places where you can rest. Sit quietly at a lakeside, in the forest, in a meadow, or in a garden. Many people consider nature a place for recreation, where the everyday burdens fall away. It is now quiet on the outside. What about the inside—of your head? Generally, the mind is racing. Thoughts revolve around problems; we worry, and create drama. This mental restlessness is perceived distinctly when the external distractions and activities cease. I would like to introduce you to an exercise that helps to achieve inner peace.

Body Scan–Mood Check

You can perform this exercise at any time. Sit or lie down comfortably, close your eyes, and switch to your »program of sensations.« This switches off the mental activity, which continuously comments, judges, and criticizes. It is an exercise in self-observation by feeling without mental judgment.

The Body Scan

After closing your eyes shift your focus first toward the sounds around you. What do you hear inside the room and from the outside?

What do you see (with the eyes closed: light, intense colors)?

Tension? Pain?

Ask yourself: how does my body feel on the ground/chair? Which areas of the body are in contact with the ground or the chair? Do I feel tension, pain, or am I free of discomfort? Slowly scan your entire body.

Move your attention from head to toe. Check if there are areas of your body that feel uncomfortable or painful. Scan the entire body for possible discomfort. If you encounter a painful or tense spot, for example, your neck, stay with it for a while and breathe into the area. After a while, continue with your scan. If you find yourself to be free of discomfort, gratefully dwell and marvel at this state of well-being.

Cold? Warm?

Scan your body again, this time observing the temperature.

Do you feel cold or have cold areas? Or do you feel excess heat in some areas? Limit yourself to mere observation and remain in the sphere of sensations. Can you feel the warmth in your chest extending all the way

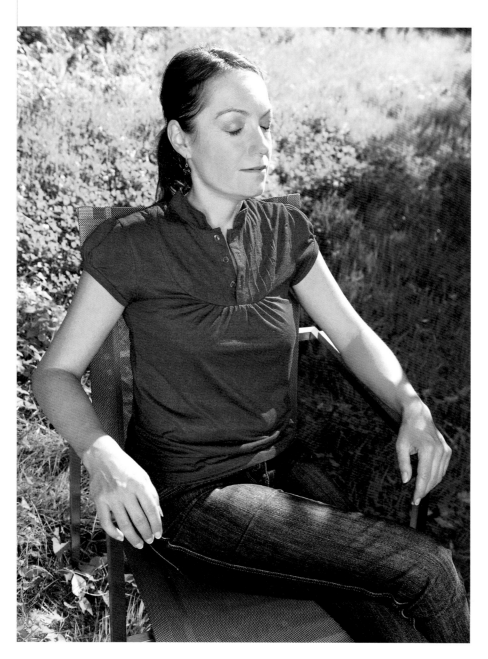

to your finger tips? Can you feel a tingling sensation on the palms and backs of your hands? If your hands are cold, feel the sensations inside you. Can you feel the warmth radiating from your abdomen into your thighs, calves, all the way to the tips of your toes? Can you feel a tingling sensation on the soles of your feet, toes, and tips of your toes?

Does your entire body feel comfortable? Not excessively cold or excessively hot? Rekindle gratefulness. If you felt cold areas, take a warm hand or foot soak later to restore your protective temperature shield.

Physical Needs?
- Check your needs
- Are you tired and want to sleep (see power nap p. 63)?
- Do you need to move?
- Do you have to eliminate (bladder/colon)?
- Are you hungry, thirsty, or full?

What is Your Mental–Emotional Condition Now?
This is a brief excursion into your mental-emotional condition. A few seconds are sufficient to imagine opening a big drawer, to acknowledge its contents, and to close it again.

◄ You can do the body scan–mood check any time: just close your eyes and feel your inner self.

How are My Family Relations?

- Father, mother, partner, children, and siblings? (Simply check, if relations are harmonious, indifferent, or burdened by conflicts.)

How is My Work Situation?

- Tension between myself and co-workers, boss, clients?
- Important contracts, concerns, »areas« that are unfinished business?
- Financial difficulties?
- Or does everything run smoothly, the »basics« are functioning?

How Do I Feel Personally?

- Health?
- Living conditions: do I like where I live?
- Do I feel comfortable at work?
- Do I feel comfortable with my partner?
- Do I follow my vision of life? Have I gone astray?

Mood Check

How do you feel right now? What do you feel?

Open the Drawer, Close the Drawer

At first you may find this exercise odd. Maybe you have tried not to think of an unpleasant issue and it keeps sneaking back into your mind. Open the the drawer, look inside, and close it. The more often you try this, the better it works. Our subconscious responds well to images. Concerns and problems do not disappear but

Which attributes apply to me right now?

Astounded	Fulfilled	Anxious	Nervous
Happy	Safe	Hopeless	Paralyzed
Well	Surprised	Angry	Discouraged
Moved	Enthusiastic	Impatient	Confused
Trusting	Emotional	Aggravated	Awkward
Optimistic	Content	Disconcerted	Hesitant
Inspired	Blessed	Concerned	Frustrated
Proud	Hopeful	Worried	Sad
Strong	Grateful	Lonely	Helpless
Relieved		Disappointed	

for the moment they are conscient and stored away in the drawer. You do not have to invest energy to suppress your thoughts. This frees your mind to perceive the actual moment.

If you end up mulling over an issue and worry again, realize the effects of these thoughts on your body. Maybe your son is on a trip in a foreign country and you do not know exactly where he is and how he is doing. Gradually your heartbeat accelerates, your neck swells, the stomach feels uneasy, and your hands get cold. When you keep checking yourself, you will notice how the negative thoughts and your worry cycle »poison« your body. One moment ago you felt relaxed and safe, nothing was wrong. As soon as you hop on the roundabout of worries you produce

neurosubstances that can damage your organs and your immunity.

Stay with Your Senses

This exercise demonstrates the results of constant worries and negative thoughts. You decide when to close the drawer again. You can repeat to yourself a specific phrase, for example »I wish the best for you and I trust that you are in good hands.«

This may help you to let go. In this very moment there is nothing you can do for your son. You should receive and enjoy whatever life offers you right now. The point of this exercise is the realization of your current worries. By identifying issues, the vague internal restlessness is dispelled. It is important to stay with the senses. Do not comment and judge. This is a

KNOWLEDGE

Remaining Silent

In religious institutions, a combination of fasting and remaining silent is practiced. Even when you do not wish to give up speaking completely while fasting, it is advisable to avoid superficial babbling. It is preferable to choose words that come from the heart, from the internal quiet space with a personal meaning or to write in a diary. If you fast with a group, arrange for a silent hike or agree on certain hours of the day when everyone remains silent. I like to remain silent during my fasts. In our clinic, we provide guests who would like to remain silent with a button stating »I remain silent.« This clarifies their silence to the other guests and does not force them to break the silence in order to explain themselves.

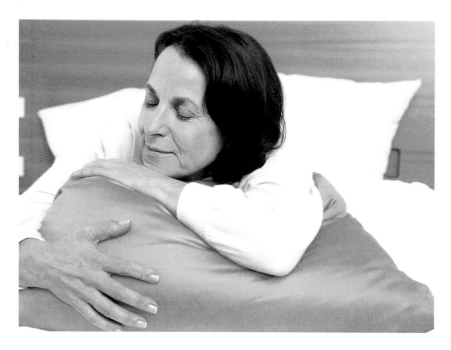

▲ During the fast you should take plenty of rest. Lie down when you are tired.

great exercise to experience the here and now and receive life's offerings to the full.

Relaxing

There are many relaxation techniques. Which technique you choose depends on your personal preferences. Prior athletic activities or exercises facilitate relaxation. Take the space and time everyday while you are fasting to come to rest. The fasting clinics offer various relaxation techniques, including yoga (see pp. 65–69) or the tried and tested autogenic techniques. Dr. Schulz, from Berlin, Germany, derived autogenic training from self-hypnosis. It is based on the following six autosuggestions:

- »I am calm«
- »My entire body feels heavy« (the feeling of heaviness originates in the relaxation of muscle tension)
- »My body feels warm« (the relaxation of the vascular muscles causes an increase in blood circulation)
- »I am breathing calmly«
- »My heart is beating calmly«
- »My solar plexus is warm«

Mental activities are reduced when a person consciously experiences bodily sensations.

Sleep When You Are Tired

Our energy level fluctuates. In the course of the day there are physiological energetic ups and downs.

Approximately every 4 hours our energy decreases, which causes us to feel really tired, and sometimes we cannot help but close our eyes. If we had the opportunity at that time to rest and give in to the tiredness, we would fall asleep. During our day-to-day working activities we often banish emerging weariness by drinking coffee.

While fasting, you can and should follow the physical signs and rest when you are tired. Drinking coffee is a no-no during the fast. You may notice the cycles of tiredness more frequently and distinctly during the fast. You can use the opportunity and train your ability to take a brief but revitalizing nap (1–20 minutes), a power nap. The body learns to take brief naps during the day in order to recharge the energy. This ability is very useful in everyday life.

KNOWLEDGE

Power Nap

- Please use a period of the day when you feel tired or feel the common after-meal fatigue for the following exercises. They work best if you have not had any coffee or tea.
- As soon as you feel heavy tiredness and have the opportunity, lie down. Some people prefer to lie on their stomachs; choose whichever position works best for you.
- Before you fall asleep, memorize the exact time when you want to wake up.
- Make sure that nothing disturbs you during the exercise (e.g., telephone).
- Ask someone to keep an eye on you and make sure to wake you up after 10 to 15 minutes. You want to prevent falling into a long, deep sleep.
- When you wake up, get up right away. Wake yourself up with some brief exercises or by washing your face with cold water. Try to re-enter your daily activities immediately. While fasting, this means, for example, going for a walk.

If you practice this exercise regularly, preferably once a day, you will soon become able to master this power nap. Some patience is required while practicing. Do not give up if it does not work right away or every time. And please do not try to force a power nap. This would violate a natural process and provoke an adverse reaction.

Movement

When properly dosed, physical activity has a positive impact on all systems of the human body, especially on respiration and blood circulation. It promotes faster, deeper breathing, while simultaneously activating the heart. Blood is moved faster through the large and small vessels, resulting in increased gaseous exchange and cell nutrition (supply of oxygen and nutrients, removal of carbon dioxide and metabolic waste). Blood flow into all tissues as well as their metabolism is encouraged, like a fire by bellows. In addition to these general effects of movement, there are specific effects that are of particular importance while fasting, including:

- maintenance/increase of muscle performance, including the cardiac muscle;
- avoiding the loss of proteins due to immobility;
- increased acid exhalation through the lungs and increased oxygen intake by the muscle cells;
- stimulation of fat burning;

KNOWLEDGE

Every Breath is a Massage for the Abdominal Organs

The lungs would only be two unmoving pouches if they were not attached to the diaphragm. This tent-like muscle, stretched between thorax and abdominal cavity, is lowered during inhalation and lifted during exhalation. When breathing freely, this causes a massage of the abdominal organs (intestines, stomach, pancreas, kidneys), which are held in place from below by the pelvic bones. During inhalation the diaphragm contracts and pushes into the abdominal cavity, which squeezes all abdominal organs, especially the digestive organs, including stomach, liver, gallbladder, pancreas, intestines, and also kidneys and spleen. This motion presses the depleted blood out of the organs. When the diaphragm returns to its original position during exhalation, the organs expand again and suck in blood that is rich in oxygen and nutrients. Regarding blood flow, inhalation and exhalation are for the abdominal organs like ebb and flow, detoxifying and nourishing.

This persistent stimulating massage is a gift of nature and can be intensified by physical activity and proper breathing exercises that cause deeper and faster respiration.

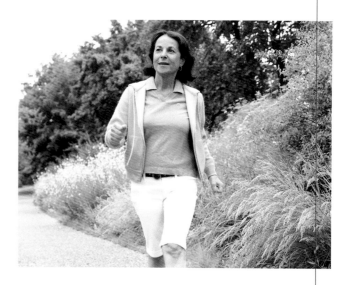

In popular literature, the diaphragm is sometimes called the second heart. Why is that? It produces suction through negative pressure. It does so first during inhalation in the thorax, which results in the lungs filling with air. During exhalation it creates negative pressure in the abdominal cavity, which exerts suction onto the lower extremities and helps to return all fluids toward the heart.

- weight reduction and stabilization of the normal weight;
- production of body heat, replacing the heat lost through the missing digestive processes;
- improved feeling of well-being and self-esteem.

Physical movement stimulates not only blood flow and respiration but also the organs of elimination, which increases elimination and regeneration processes, including:

- stimulation of kidney activity, supporting the elimination of acids through increased renal perfusion, if an adequate amount of liquid is consumed (1–2.5 L per day);
- stimulation of intestinal activity through massage by the diaphragm;
- stimulation of lung activity, including the elimination of acids in the form of carbon dioxide and other gases;
- stimulation of cutaneous perfusion and active perspiration.

Helpful Yoga Exercises

In the following I will introduce some yoga exercises to you that are especially valuable during a fast. I will briefly explain their primary effects. Take your time to familiarize yourself with the sequence of the exercises. You should perform these exercises in a relaxed and undisturbed setting. Do not take the movements beyond your comfort zone.

Exercise to Release Gas

This exercise massages and activates the large intestine, moves gas or air along the entire intestines, removes congestions of the intestinal lymph, activates intestinal peristalsis, and cleanses the lungs through intensified exhalation.

Lie full-length on your back, both arms alongside your body:
- During inhalation, move your extended arms above your head (Figure 1).
- During exhalation, bend your right knee and pull it toward your torso (Figure 2).
  - At the same time, bring your head toward the knee.
  - Wrap your hands around the knee.
- During inhalation, place the extended arms behind your head and stretch the right leg again.

- During exhalation, bend your left knee and pull it toward the torso.
  - At the same time, bring your head toward the knee.
  - Wrap your hands around the knee.
- During inhalation, place the extended arms behind your head and stretch the left leg again.
- During exhalation, bend both knees and pull them toward the torso (Figure 3).
  - At the same time, bring your head toward the knees.
  - Wrap your hands around the knees.

Repeat the entire cycle three to five times.

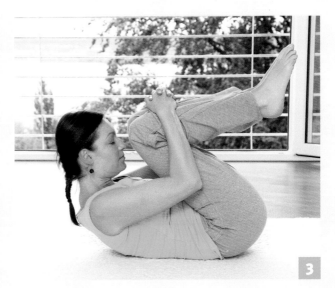

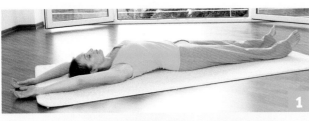

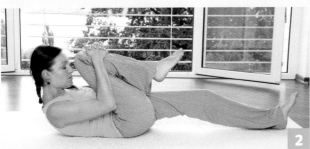

The Crocodile

The crocodile releases tension in the muscles of the back and in the bony structure of the spine. It stretches the sides of the torso, relaxes the diaphragm, and opens space for respiration. Lie full-length on your back, bend your knees, and place your feet flat on the ground. Extend your arms and place them above your head (Figure 1).

- During exhalation, slowly lower your knees to the left while turning your head to the right (Figure 2).
- During inhalation, return knees and head to their initial position.
- During exhalation, slowly lower your knees to the right while turning your head to the left (Figure 3).

Repeat the entire cycle five to seven times.

It is important that you perform this exercise slowly, steadily, and synchronized with your breath. Allow your knees to drop only to the point where you perceive a pleasant stretch.

Accept possible blockages or pain as natural limits and move within the pain-free range.

Letting Your Breath Flow

Remain lying on your back, gently place your hands on your abdomen, and observe your inhalations and exhalations. Your breath flows well if your abdomen rises during inhalation and falls during exhalation. Your breath is too shallow if you cannot perceive any motion of the abdomen, either during inhalation or during exhalation.

The following exercise demonstrates how to intensify your breath. Inhale and exhale as usual but hold your breath for a few seconds after exhalation. What happens when you inhale again? You are breathing deeper and slower. This is the type of breathing you want to attain. Deep relaxation can only be achieved when breathing is deep and relaxed.

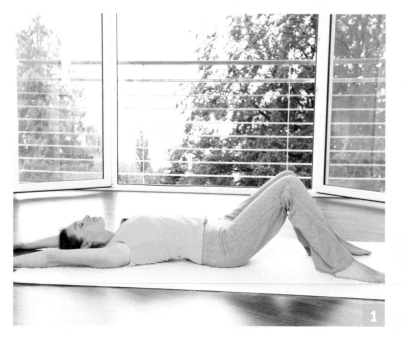

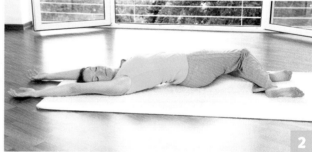

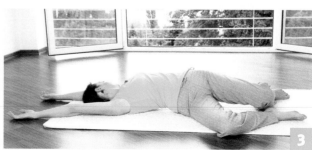

Yogic Breathing

Natural breathing, or yogic breathing, is the basis of practicing yoga. I will now introduce three breathing spaces: the abdominal space, the thoracic space, and the clavicular area. The contraction of the diaphragm initiates inhalation. When the diaphragm contracts it flattens and the air first enters the lower tips of the lungs. From there, the breath enters the thorax, noticeable through the extension of the costal arch. Finally, the breath fills the upper section of the lungs, the clavicular area. When practicing yogic breathing, you can visualize filling the three breathing spaces during inhalation and emptying them during exhalation.

Lie on your back with the legs extended; rest on the floor, place your hands gently on your abdomen, and keep your eyes closed.

Imagine how air flows into the lower tips of the lungs when you inhale. Feel how your abdomen rises and imagine (during the same inhalation) how the air enters the chest. Feel how the cos-

tal arch extends, while you complete the inhalation by letting the air flow into the upper part of the lungs, the clavicular area. When you exhale, you first empty the lower tips of the lungs, followed by the thorax, and finish with the clavicular area. Continue to breathe this way, inhaling and exhaling deeply.

The Cat

This exercise has a relaxing effect on all organs and encourages the blood flow to the organs. It releases internal and muscular tension and brings more flexibility to the spine. Go down on your hands and knees, the »on all fours« position, as shown in the pictures:

- During exhalation, lower your head between your arms and arch your back upwardly, the cat's arched back (Figure 1).
- During inhalation, lift your head and stretch your back as far as possible (Figure 2).

Repeat this cycle five to seven times.

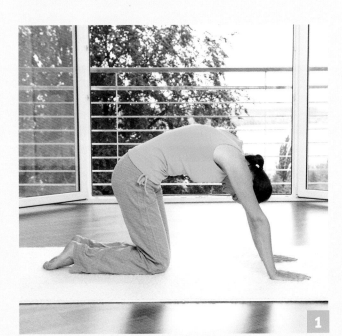

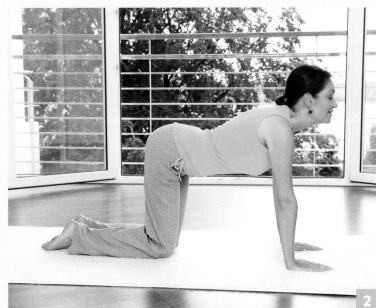

Child's Pose

This is an ideal position to relax the back. In addition, it stimulates the blood flow to the head and stretches the sciatic nerve.

Sit down on your heels and place the knees apart; rest your torso on your thighs and your forehead on the floor (see figure below); extend your arms above your head and place them on the floor or rest them next to your body. Alter the position if necessary to make sure it feels relaxed and comfortable to you, for example, by placing a pillow under your forehead.

- Hold this position for 10 to 15 relaxed breaths.
- Then, during inhalation, return your upper body and head to the upright position, let your arms hang down loosely, and remain in this position for another 10 to 15 breaths.

Alternate Nostril Breathing

Alternate nostril breathing balances the assembling and disassembling metabolic principles, cleanses the entire system, and strengthens the nerves.

Sit in the lotus position, legs crossed and back erect, on the floor, or sit on a chair with your back erect.

- Close your right nostril with your right thumb (Figure 1).
- Inhale and exhale through the left nostril.
- Continue breathing through your left nostril for 2 minutes.
- Now close the left nostril with the ring and little finger of the right hand (Figure 2), removing the thumb from the right nostril.
- Inhale and exhale through the right nostril.
- Continue breathing through your right nostril for 2 minutes.

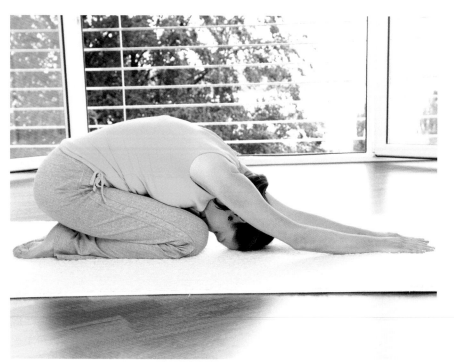

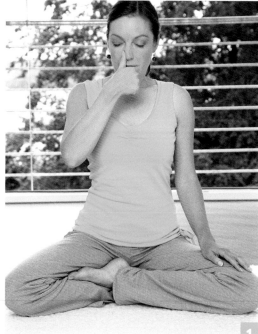

The Cleansing Yogic Breathing—Sitali Pranayama

This breathing exercise cleanses the blood and is cooling. Sit on the floor in the lotus position, legs crossed and back erect, or sit on a chair with your back erect:

- Form a »U« with your tongue, as shown in the picture, that is surrounded by your lips (right figure)
- During inhalation, draw the air in through the »U« formed by your tongue (it produces a metallic taste).
- During exhalation, close your mouth and let the air exit through your nose.

Continue for 15 to 20 breaths.

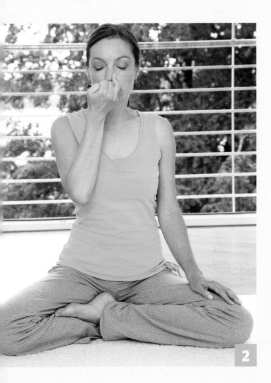

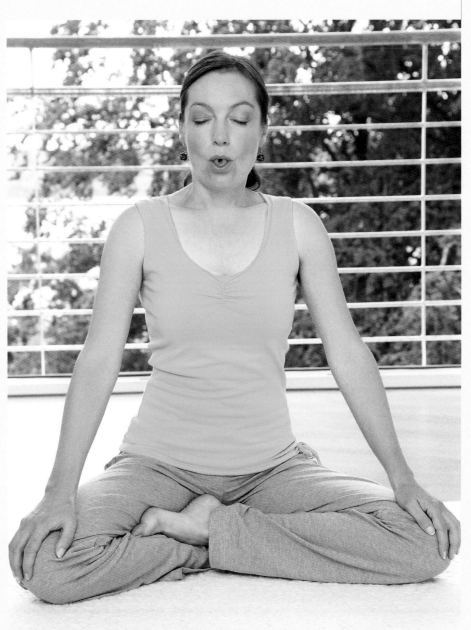

Boosting Elimination (»Detox«)

»Detox,« purification, and cleansing are terms that are usually associated with fasting. I will now introduce some methods to you that stimulate the organs of elimination, which is vital during the fast. These methods include colonic irrigation, an unjustifiably dreaded procedure.

What is part of a detoxification program?
- Clearing of possible infectious locations (e.g., teeth, nasal sinuses, urinary tract, and colon)
- Stimulation of the organs of elimination, including gut, kidneys, lungs, liver, gallbladder, and skin (see table)
- Mental–emotional eliminations (fears, conflicts, and emotional needs, as well as acknowledging feelings of powerlessness and processing them properly)

The first step is the clearing of infectious locations to relieve the immune system. This includes a visit to the dentist. Infections at the roots of dead teeth, called granulomas, are located with the help of x-ray images. This cluster of anaerobic bacteria is the size of a pinhead and may cause fever, fatigue, and non-specific complaints. After tooth restoration by a dentist, the general condition can improve

rapidly. The same set of symptoms can be produced by chronic sinusitis or chronic urinary infections.

It may be a bold statement to call the colon an infectious focus, nevertheless, an imbalanced intestinal flora is a burden to the immune system. Compared with the size of a tooth granuloma, the number of harmful intestinal bacteria is many times higher. The following steps of detoxification refer to the stimulation of the elimination processes, including physical and mental–emotional elimination, as illustrated in the following table.

Hot Liver Pack

The hot liver pack (e.g., hot-water bottle on a thin moist cloth) stimulates liver activity, which is usually applied for 30 to 60 minutes during the midday rest.

While on a Buchinger Amplius fast, a hot liver pack during the midday rest is a must. The fasting person lies in bed with a hot-water bottle at his/her feet (when they are cold). The person's torso lies on a narrow blanket that is spread out crossways. A small cloth is soaked with water, wrung out, and placed on the liver area (one

hand's width to the right of the navel on the costal arch). The hot-water bottle is placed flat on the moist cloth (do not forget to let the air out!) and the blanket is wrapped around the torso.

If you want to apply the hot liver pack yourself, you should first fill the water bottles with hot water, prepare the moist cloth, and put on a tight T-shirt. Lie down in bed, place one hot-water bottle at your feet, lift the T-shirt and place the moist cloth and the second hot-water bottle on the liver area, pull the tight shirt over the water bottle to hold it in place and cover yourself with the bedspread. This produces a warm blissful state that almost makes you want to purr.

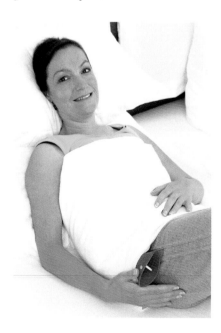

Detoxification—various techniques for the stimulation of the organs of elimination

Liver/bile	Intestines	Skin	Kidneys	Lungs
Desired effects				
▪ Stimulating bile production and bile flow ▪ Promoting liver perfusion	▪ Eliminating content of intestines ▪ Activating peristalsis ▪ Restoring a healthy intestinal flora	▪ Stimulating cutaneous perfusion ▪ Promoting perspiration ▪ Supplying with substances through the skin	▪ Stimulating renal perfusion ▪ Eliminating acids ▪ Eliminating water and metabolic waste products	▪ Exhaling acids (carbon dioxide) ▪ Oxygen intake ▪ Producing a suction effect for fluids from the lower extremities ▪ Abdominal massage through diaphragmatic breathing, stimulating bowel movement
Helpful measures				
▪ Hot liver pack ▪ Healing plants: rosemary, boldo ▪ Various measures, including acupuncture, yoga asanas, and enzymes ▪ Various fruits and vegetables, e.g., artichokes, olive oil	▪ Promote diaphragmatic activity through breathing and exercise ▪ Laxatives: teas (senna), castor oil, sauerkraut juice ▪ Glauber's salt, Epsom salts ▪ Colonic irrigation, high colonics ▪ Natural fillers, e.g., plums, figs, flax seed, fibers ▪ Colon massage (also self-massage) ▪ Restoring the intestinal flora ▪ Whole foods	▪ Physical activity (active perspiration) ▪ Dry brushing ▪ Hydro/Kneipp therapy, warm baths, sauna, steam bath, warm air baths (passive perspiration) ▪ Sun bathing ▪ Massage ▪ Healing plants, e.g., Hamamelis ▪ Oil application	▪ Drinking water ▪ Physical activities (quicken circulation) ▪ Eating low-sodium diet, fruits and vegetables, e.g., onions, leeks ▪ Healing plants, e.g., birch, linden, cherry, stinging nettle ▪ Wraps, compresses ▪ Various: swimming, reflexotherapy of the feet, TCM	▪ Physical activities (accelerating respiratory rate and depth) ▪ Breathing therapy, respiratory massage, yoga (pranayama) ▪ Healing plants, e.g., eucalyptus, menthol, pine, thyme

Moist heat penetrates the body deeper than dry heat, which produces two results:

- The moist heat and the lying position cause intense liver perfusion, which stimulates its detoxification and metabolic function.
- The person relaxes, restores his/her energy, and can compensate for a possible sleep deficit.

Intestinal Hygiene during the Fast

The stimulation of intestinal elimination is drastically reduced when a person only takes in juices and broth. Even so, small amounts of digestive juices and bile are produced, the mucous membrane peels away, and intestinal bacteria and epithelial cells must be removed. Experience shows that regular colonic irrigation increases well-being and performance. In addition, gastrointestinal complaints and headaches can be avoided.

Glauber's Salt

On the morning of the first day of the fast, ca. 20 to 40 g Glauber's salt (sodium sulfate) are dissolved in 500 to 750 mL of water and taken within 20 minutes of mixing.

Generally, the following dosage guidelines apply:

- Prepare the Glauber's salt solution:
  - 20 g Glauber's salt if you tend to diarrhea and/or are underweight;
  - 30 g Glauber's salt for people with normal weight and regular bowel movement;
  - 40 g Glauber's salt if you tend to be constipated and/or are overweight;
  - the Glauber's salt is dissolved in 500 to 750 mL of warm water.
- You can prepare a »taste improving« beverage, containing 2 tablespoons raspberry syrup and 1 tablespoon lemon juice dissolved in a glass of cold water (caution: diabetics omit the raspberry syrup and only take the lemon juice!).
- Alternate between drinking a glass of Glauber's salt solution and a few sips of the »taste improver.« Drink everything within 15 to 20 minutes.
- Treat yourself to two cups of peppermint tea, 1 hour after finishing the Glauber's salt solution; it stimulates the bile production and calms the intestines. Continue by drinking plenty of water.

The osmotic effect of the Glauber's salt leads to the retention of large amounts of fluid within the intestinal lumen. This fluid expands the walls of the colon, which responds with elimination.

Colonic Irrigation

People with fasting experience often simply know the proper moment for colonic irrigation. When fasting for the first time, you should follow the rule of cleansing the colon every other day. To some people this is »non-natural,« to some plain »awful,« and others complain about »medi-

---

KNOWLEDGE

Gently Easing into the Fast

For some people it is advisable to gently ease into the fast and skip the Glauber's salt. Indications for this approach include the following:

- Sensitive gastrointestinal tract (e.g., gallbladder disorders, tendency to suffer from gastritis and/or diarrhea)
- Low blood pressure and »low-energy-level« constitution
- Tendency for headaches and migraine
- Disorders of the lumbar spine
- Exhaustion

In these cases, a milder type of laxative is chosen (e.g., laxative tea from the pharmacy) or colonic irrigation, which can be repeated 3 days straight, can be given. The return to a regular diet must also begin cautiously.

KNOWLEDGE

Colonic Irrigation—Beyond the Fasting Period

Beyond the fasting period, colonic irrigation is recommended if one or several of the following symptoms are present:
- Flatulence, abdominal discomfort
- Changes in the shape of the abdomen
- Coated tongue, impressions of the teeth on the tongue
- Halitosis (bad breath)
- Fatigue, especially in the morning and after eating
- Restlessness at night, sleeping disorders
- Lack of appetite in the morning

These symptoms indicate that you should reconsider your eating habits and lifestyle.

Contraindications include:
- Acute appendicitis or inflammation of other abdominal organs
- Acute diverticulitis

eval medical punishment«! Intestinal hygiene is still a taboo subject and is rarely practiced by people who do not experience any discomforts. Well, brushing your teeth is also »non-natural« but necessary due to modern nutrition. Every home medicine chest should contain colonic irrigation supplies. Colonic irrigation is a simple, effective, and yet inexpensive way to stop infections, eliminate indigestion, and even bring bouts of inflammatory diseases, for example, inflammation of joints, to a halt.

Be Cautious!

In spite of all the positive effects, you must remember that colonic irrigation can dehydrate and flush out some body minerals. Therefore, it is important to drink plenty of water and watch the mineral supply to the body. Vegetable broth and juices (outside the fasting period larger amounts may be consumed) are important providers of these substances. Minerals can also be taken in the form of tablets. In case of hemorrhoids, the irrigation nozzle needs to be well lubricated and inserted slowly and carefully.

Conducting Colonic Irrigation

Where? In a quiet place, in the bathroom when doing it by yourself.

How Long? Ca. 20 to 30 minutes altogether.

When? In the morning, or in the evening before going to bed; otherwise, during a relaxed time of the day.

How? Either a nurse gives the colonic irrigation or you do it yourself. If a nurse gives the colonic irrigation, you lie on a plastic covering on your bed. If you do it by yourself, the knee-elbow position is recommended:
- Fill the colonic irrigation bag with 1 to 1.5 L tepid water (37°C).
- Open the flow control valve, allow air bubbles to exit, and close the valve.
- Hang the colonic irrigation bag from a door knob or a towel rack.
- Lubricate the colonic irrigation nozzle with some Vaseline.
- Adopt the knee-elbow position (meaning to support yourself with knees and elbows) and use one hand to insert the nozzle into the rectum. If this is too uncomfortable for you, you may adopt any other position, as long as your body remains below the irrigation bag for the water to follow the differential into the colon.
- Open the valve to begin the process.
- Once the entire amount of water has entered the colon, shut the valve and remove the nozzle.
- If possible, hold the water for 1 to 3 minutes.

After the initial spontaneous elimination, the effects of the colonic irrigation can be increased through a colon self-massage or rapid movements of the abdominal wall.

Colon Hydrotherapy (High Colonics)

Colon hydrotherapy is a procedure in which the colonic irrigation bag is replaced by a device that regulates continuous influx of tepid water into the colon as well as the water removal. Consider it a sort of high-tech colonic irrigation! During the procedure, an experienced therapist massages the abdomen and ensures maximum colon elimination.

Colon Massage

The colon massage, put together by P. Vogler, is very well suited for the stimulation of intestinal activity. It has proven successful not only during a fast but also in cases of chronic constipation. This technique also expedites the effects of colonic irrigation. Lie on your back in a comfortable position and relax. Make sure your hands are warm and begin to massage your colon. You locate and massage five areas, one by one. In these areas, the colon is attached to the posterior abdominal wall and there is a 90% chance of properly locating it.

At each of the five sites you do as follows: during exhalation, you press with both your hands down into the abdomen and perform a pushing motion toward the next site. Ideally, at the beginning of the motion you move your hands slightly against the main direction of movement to prevent excessive pull on the abdominal skin. Repeat this motion for 2 to 4 minutes at each site.

Maintain continuous contact between your hands and your abdomen, even when your hands are at rest and not exerting any pressure.

This is how to locate the five sites (Figures 1 to 5):

1. Cecum point: on an imaginary line between navel and the ASIS (anterior superior iliac spine), ca. two to three fingers' width superior to the ASIS toward the navel.
2. Ascendant point: below the right costal arch.
3. Lineal point: below the left costal arch.
4. Descendant point: mirroring the first point, on the left side.
5. Sigma point: right above the pubic bone, in the center of the torso. The bladder is located directly underneath and should therefore be emptied before the treatment.

At the end, you perform some clockwise circles with your flat right hand on your abdomen around the navel. This treatment takes 15 to 20 minutes if performed as directed above.

Dry Brushing/Rubbing and Oil Application

Dry brushing of the skin, also called brush massage, stimulates the perfu-

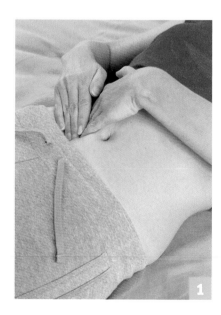
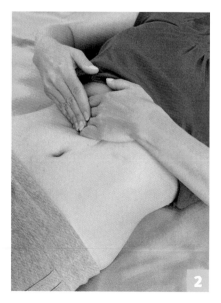

sion and metabolic activities of the skin. This improves skin nourishment as well as skin cleansing. This technique also has a balancing effect on blood pressure. Due to its skin renewing, restoring, and toning effects, dry brushing additionally offers some cosmetic qualities.

The procedure is easy to follow: brush in circles or straight lines toward the heart, generally, following the left-yields-to-right rule.

This means that you brush the right leg before you brush the left leg, brush the right arm before you brush the left arm, brush the abdomen clockwise, gently brush the chest, and finish by brushing the back.

KNOWLEDGE

Nasal Rinsing

Regular nasal rinsing is recommended not only during the fasting period, but also as an everyday routine. You can prevent colds, clear up your nose when it is congested by colds or hay fever, diminish inflammations of nasal or frontal sinuses, and provide relief for house-dust allergies. In yoga practice, the neti pot is used to cleanse the nose and the sinuses of mucus and inhaled substances. Pharmacies provide nasal douches that follow the same yogic principle. In nose rinsing, an isotonic saline solution is used that you may either purchase or prepare yourself: dissolve 9 g pharmaceutically cleansed salt in 1 L of boiled water. Use a tepid solution for the nasal rinsing. Never use water without salt!

Subsequent to the brushing it is recommended to take a hot–cold alternating shower and to oil your skin. It is best to use high-quality organic grade oils or lotions, apply them generously, and rub until absorbed. This procedure is also recommended as part of the daily body care.

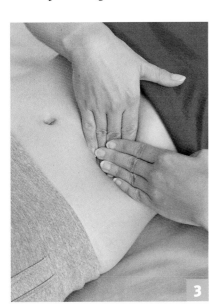

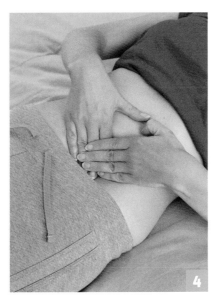

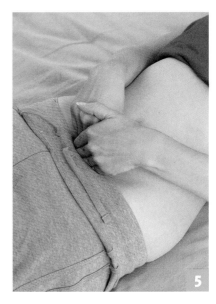

Adjuvant Therapies

IV

Since Dr. Otto Buchinger's time, three generations later, the adjuvant therapies have evolved. As a result of globalization, we are familiar not only with conventional massages but also with treatments from other cultures, including respiratory therapy, hydrotherapy, Kneipp therapies and osteopathy from Europe; acupuncture, acupressure, and *tuina* from China; or ayurvedic massages and *chi nei tsang*.

During a fast, the proper dosage of therapies is of particular importance, that is, the stimulus has to match the individual ability to process and respond to the stimulus. The basic biological rule is as follows: weak stimulation affects nothing. Proper stimulation facilitates physical reactions. Excessive stimulation inhibits reactions or has a detrimental effect. Most fasting clinics offer the therapies that will be described in this section, plus numerous others.

Massage

During the course of a fast, we prefer partial massages of the painful areas or full body massages. In combination with specifically tailored exercises, they serve to maintain or restore mobility. Owing to their relaxing and circulation-enhancing effects, as well as the emotional value of therapeutic touch and skin contact, massages are very popular. Allow yourself to rest for half an hour after the massage, taking full advantage of its resonance and giving the body the opportunity for a healing response!

Hydrotherapy

All types of water applications (hydrotherapy) may be utilized in individualized dosages, including Kneipp affusions, ablutions, compresses, wraps, and even medicinal baths. However, thermal stimulation must be applied with great caution. Cold applications are beneficial only if the body is able to respond properly and restore warmth right afterward. While fasting, people tend to be sensitive to cold, because they lack the heat produced by digestive processes. Warm therapies, such as sauna, baths, and water treading (or »Kneipping«) are beneficial, but should be of limited duration to go easy on circulation.

Breathing Therapy

Fasting is an ideal situation to release restricted respiration. Emptying the gastrointestinal tract and general weight reduction leads to improved diaphragmatic mobility. The yogic pranayama exercises, in particular, demonstrate a maximum three-phase expansion of the respiratory motion during inhalation and maximum pulmonary deflation during exhalation. Restrictive clothing, false posture, and lack of exercise can limit our respiratory functions, and so can mental–emotional factors. Who has not experienced the tight sensation in the chest during tense or frightening situations? Respiration automatically adapts to physical and psychological situations. If this automatic adaptation fails to function properly, techniques of respiratory therapy will exercise and restore these mechanisms. Respiratory therapy or »Atemtherapie« according to Glaser or Middendorf acts primarily on the respiratory dysfunctions caused by psychological disorders. Respiratory exercises on the physical level of stretching muscles and fibers deepen and regulate respiration. Both methods complement each other well. The therapist's hand exerts a certain amount of pressure by resting on the affected areas while following the breathing rhythm and balancing energy fields. This pressure can loosen the blockages and restore the regular respiratory function.

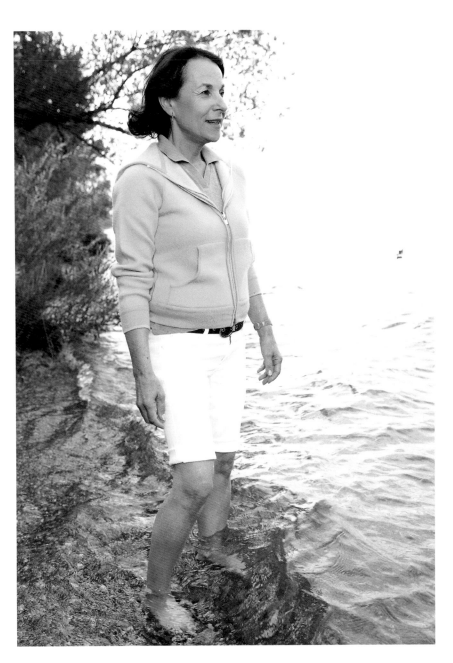

The Roeder Method

For the Roeder therapy, the nasal mucous membranes are stimulated with the use of cotton swabs. Since he fell gravely ill as a result of tonsillitis, at a time without antibiotics, Dr. Otto Buchinger considered the method, developed by the Wuppertal physician Heinrich Roeder, essential while fasting.

The cotton swab is dipped into a mixture of diluted essential oils. The cotton swab is then inserted into the nostril until it meets with the posterior pharyngeal wall. This stimulates the reflex zones of the nasal mucous membranes, which results in intense perfusion. In addition, the physician may aspirate the palatal tonsils and wipe off the pharyngeal tonsils.

This application is especially suited for patients who frequently suffer from colds. During a fast, the application provides additional general circulatory and metabolic stimulation.

Phytotherapy

In addition to individually prescribed medicinal substances, drinking tea is an option of phytotherapeutic treatment, including the following:

◄ I find Kneipp's water treading in Lake Constance superbly refreshing.

- Anise-fennel-caraway for flatulence
- Peppermint for nausea
- Stinging nettle against water retention
- Black or green tea for low blood pressure
- Ginger for sensitivity to cold

People with sensitive stomachs should avoid »red« teas (e.g., hibiscus, rosehip) and drink »blond« teas, including linden and chamomile.

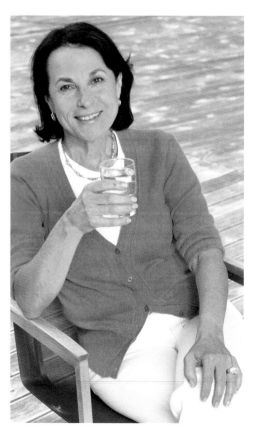

Care

V

People who are on a fast must be cared for, even if they are experienced in fasting. The best how-to book cannot replace human care. I do not mind repeating it again: it is not advisable to fast without expert care and support!

- Members of a religious order, who are experienced in fasting, are supported at times by another nun. The everyday life in an order is very structured and the spiritual dimension is omnipresent and therefore conducive to fasting.
- In a fasting group, the fasting counselor takes care of the group members, preferably with a physician on the sidelines.
- In a fasting clinic, care is ideal and all adjuvant therapies that act synergistically are readily available (e.g., in the clinics in Überlingen/Lake Constance, Germany and Marbella, Spain).

(For addresses of clinics see p. IX.)

Fasting Beverages

VI

Drink plenty is a fasting motto. You should drink ca. 1.5 to 2 L of water or calorie-free herbal tea per day. Plenty of fluids dilute elimination products, for example, uric acid, and stimulate kidney functions. Usually food supplies a large portion of fluids, therefore, while fasting, you must drink larger amounts. Fasting beverages and supplements should be freshly prepared and natural, just like the food right before and after the fast. Buchinger Amplius therapeutic fasting uses the following fasting beverages:

- 250 mL of fruit or vegetable juice (freshly juiced if possible)
- 250 mL vegetable broth
- Teas, if necessary with honey (2 to 3 teaspoons in the course of the day)
- Mineral water (low in sodium, nitrate, and non-carbonated)

These beverages provide up to 250 kcal, vitamins, minerals, and secondary plant compounds per day.

The following supplements may be individually required in addition to the above-listed fasting beverages:
- Protein

- Micronutrients (minerals and vitamins)
- Essential fatty acids

Protein

Considering today's excess supply of protein, we do not see the general need to supplement protein, if an average nutritional condition is present and the fast is conducted in a methodically proper fashion. Stopping the ingestion of proteins for a limited period can even be therapeutically advantageous.

In weak and older people it may be helpful to supplement protein via natural products, such as buttermilk, yoghurt, various dairy products, or almond or soy milk (500 to 750 mL per day). This nutrition supplies »fresh«

amino acids to the body and the fasting person does not need to exclusively »recycle« the body's own proteins.

Micronutrients and Essential Fatty Acids

During a fast that lasts 2 to 4 weeks, supplementation of micronutrients is generally not required in people with a balanced nutritional condition.

Supplementation in addition to the juices and vegetable broth may be appropriate if a deficiency in vitamins and minerals is suspected or in cases of elevated demand.

In chronic diseases, micronutrients are supplied, as well as essential fatty acids in their native cis-cis form

(cold-pressed sunflower/flax seed oil), for example, in the form of the following:

- In the morning: 250 mL freshly squeezed carrot juice and 50 g low-fat curd with a teaspoon of cold-pressed sunflower oil.
- In the afternoon: 50 g low-fat curd or one yoghurt with a teaspoon of flax seed oil (blend curd/yoghurt and oil well).

Vitamin and Mineral Supplementation

Vitamin deficiency is caused either through insufficient supply (e.g., unbalanced or poor diet, especially lack of fruit, vegetables, and fresh products) or increased demand (e.g., vitamin C in smokers; vitamin B1 in alcoholics; iron, calcium, and folic acid during pregnancy and nursing). During stress and disease, there is usually a higher demand for vitamins and minerals, which must be met. If a deficiency is suspected, supplements may be given in addition to minerals and vitamins contained in the juices and vegetable broth.

It is questionable if fasting is the proper thing to do in this condition. A different form of nutritional therapy may be preferable (e.g., lacto-ovo vegetarian nutrition or, if it is tolerable, raw food diet). The balance of sodium and other minerals, such as potassium, calcium, and magnesium

FROM MY EXPERIENCES

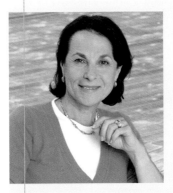

I Dilute the Fruit Juice with Water

When I fast, I tend to feel cold and have low blood pressure. Therefore, I usually drink warm beverages. I dilute the 250 mL of fruit juice with water (ca. 1 L) and drink it in small sips during the course of the day. My favorite beverage is grape juice. I sort of hoard it. After diluting it, I make sure that it will last me for the rest of the day. As an exception, I may have one or two sips of green tea to boost my circulation.

KNOWLEDGE

Dreams

You live with double intensity if you remember your dreams. Fasting is an ideal time to experience your dreams and enter into a dialogue with the subconscious.

Some tips on how to »catch« your dreams:

- Place pen and paper on your night stand.
- Concentrate and wish for a dream at night right before you go to sleep.
- Immediately write down your dream and all spontaneous associations when you wake up.
- Imagine all elements and people that are part of a dream being a possible part of you.
- Work through your dreams with the help of a professional.

is primarily regulated by the kidneys, in collaboration with hormones of the adrenal cortex. The blood concentration of these minerals remains unchanged during the fast, unless laxatives and diuretic medication were taken regularly previous to the fast. In this case mineral supplements are prescribed.

Soul Food

The emotional balance of a person is maintained by cultivating or rediscovering sources of positive emotions, including visual art, literature, music, meditation, nature, as well as human relations and spirituality. What about the »nine nutrients« for your soul (see pp. 14–17)? Utilize the fasting period for new discoveries. The abstention of unhealthy but pleasurable everyday habits is facilitated because you have the opportunity to discover sources of pleasure beyond culinary delights. Dream messages are also part of the soul dietetics.

What Brings You Joy?

Take a piece of paper and write down everything that brings you joy and pleasure, including things that you enjoyed when you were 10 or 16! It is then up to you to sort through this list and (re)activate the most important sources of pleasure. For personal or work-related reasons, many people limit their sources for pleasure to food, drink, and work, believing that »they have it all.« Furthermore, take a close look at your network of relations.

Cultivate or Vitalize Your Network of Relations

Fasting is an ideal time to take a close look at your network of relations. How is the relationship with your family, friends, and co-workers? Which relationships are vital, which are blocked or have not been maintained for a long time? Conflicts with partners, siblings, parents, and children lead to a considerable loss of emotional energy and stress. It is easier for fasting people to initiate an internal peace process. It may begin with thoughts you dedicate to that person, a letter, a phone call, or a dialogue with your diary. It is amazing how fast a relationship can be rekindled if one of the people involved opens up to it.

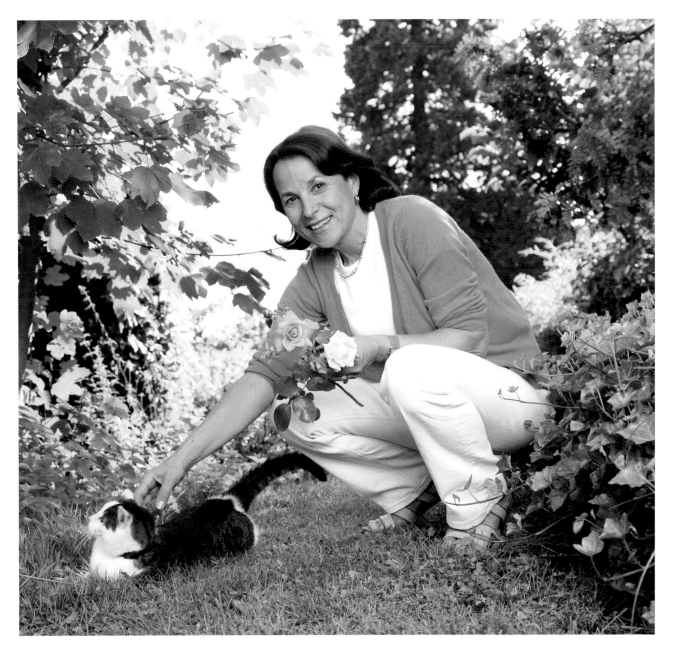

Dealing with Possible
Discomforts or Crises

I would like to give you some practical advice in the section below, about possible discomforts or even serious fasting crises and what to do about them.

Most disorders can usually be remedied by small interventions, such as rest, activities, communication to reduce fears, and naturopathic measures. A fasting crisis on the other hand is an acute condition that requires medical attention. It can frequently be considered a cleansing and healing crisis, but it could also be the result of a pre-existing condition or occur because fasting rules have not been followed.

Don't Smoke! Don't Drink Alcohol!

» Eating and fasting are incompatible and so are smoking and fasting. Smoking is a known health hazard, particularly during a fast.

After a few drags on a cigarette, the capillaries contract in a corkscrew pattern and blood flow is slowed down. This causes stasis in some parts of the capillary network. When smoking only one cigarette, it takes 1 hour for the disturbances in this system to subside. All organs and bodily functions depend on proper perfusion and must be protected from additional strain caused by toxins, such as tar and heavy metals, which are inhaled when smoking. Lead and cadmium, also involved in smoking, are heavier burdens on the person smoking and the environment than is urban air contamination.

Nicotine is a proven factor in cardiovascular diseases, which rank first in the statistics of general and death-causing diseases. Approximately 40% of all cancerous diseases could be avoided by not smoking. Lung cancer, 90% caused by smoking, has reached record highs. Have you stubbed out your cigarette yet or would you like me to continue? Here is some good news for smokers who have tried to quit smoking without success: during a fast, the withdrawal is significantly easier. Make use of the fasting period to get away from cigarettes. I know plenty of people who were able to kick this habit easily while fasting.

Alcohol also must not be consumed while fasting. Primarily in habitual drinkers, pathological changes in the nervous system and internal organs, including heart, liver, pancreas, stomach, and intestines are frequently observed. These changes can be corrected through fasting. Already the

first fasting cure produces significant improvements.

Not even one drop of alcohol is allowed during a fast because it:
- strains the liver;
- stimulates the gastric juices, which irritates the stomach and causes feelings of hunger;
- depletes vitamins;
- inhibits detoxification.

This is different for a healthy person on a regular diet. A nice glass of wine can be stimulating! The evil is in the dosage!

KNOWLEDGE

Problems during a Fast

Difficulties may arise if:
- there is a pre-existing condition;
- medication is taken that requires adjusting;
- fasting rules are not followed (e.g., drink plenty of water, balance rest and exercise, take your time to return to a regular diet);
- adequate care is unavailable.

Possible Discomforts During a Fast

» In the following section, I will list numerous possible disorders. It is, however, most unlikely that you will experience all of them; a few maybe and only temporarily.

Sensitivity to Cold
The heat production through digestive processes is absent and the production of thyroid hormones is slightly reduced. It is recommended that you dress warmly, drink warm beverages (also warm water!), take warm baths, visit the sauna, exercise your body, or fast during the warm season.

Fatigue
Fatigue appears in different degrees. It may present itself somewhere between difficulties in concentrating and apathy. There are numerous causes and matching solutions, such as the following:
- Sleep deficit and exhaustion prior to fasting can be remedied by sleep. Allow yourself plenty of rest.
- Low blood pressure can be counteracted with exercise and washing the face with cold water.
- In the case of hypoglycemia, the person should lie down and rest, keep warm, and maybe drink some

tea with honey. Slight hypoglycemia, combined with the feeling of exhaustion, may occur after physical overexertion and extended sunbathing.
- Chronic fatigue may be a sign of psychological inhibition and depression. This condition is best approached with communication, psychotherapy, or nonverbal procedures, including breathing therapy, energy balancing, or keeping a diary.

Low Blood Pressure or Dizziness
- If you feel dizzy upon rising, you should avoid any type of rushing and get up in two stages. Change from lying into a seated position and from there slowly into an upright position.

FROM MY EXPERIENCES

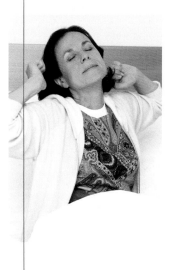

I Want to Sleep all the Time

At the beginning of my fasts, I may feel drugged with fatigue. I do not fight it but allow myself the necessary rest. When my body needs sleep, it should get it. I support the metabolic changes by taking a shower or a bath with fragrant additives or by dry brushing. After the first colonic irrigation I experience a distinct improvement. During this adjustment stage I like getting massages and dislike talking. On the third day I usually wake up feeling an energetic balance and the desire to go for a walk and inhale fresh air. I change from a hibernating groundhog into a migrating bird that can fast and simultaneously be completely active.

- In the case of low blood pressure, drink ample amounts of liquids to maintain proper blood volume and regularly practice endurance training.
- In acute dizziness, lie down immediately with elevated legs to promote blood flow back to the heart and the head.

Headache

Many coffee drinkers are plagued by headaches owing to caffeine withdrawal. Headaches are also blamed on the initial water elimination as well as general detoxification. They often disappear abruptly after thorough intestinal cleansing. Helpful in combating this headache is timely colonic irrigation, drinking ample amounts of liquids, head lymph drainage, massaging the temples with peppermint oil, lots of rest, and fresh air. Sometimes a cold pack placed on the forehead brings relief. The need to take medication arises rarely. Our insider's tip: get into fasting in stages.

Low Back Pains

Enormous strain is placed on the »hinge« between the pelvic bones and the lumbar spine. This results in degenerative changes with the corresponding muscular tension, which causes numerous complaints in this area during a fast. Dehydration, increased acid production, and possibly imbalanced mineral levels are the probable reasons for these discomforts. Heat, exercises, swimming, physical therapy, or osteopathy may be of help, as well as drinking ample amounts of liquids and supplementing minerals and alkaline substances, if applicable.

Nausea / Bile-vomiting

Fasting may cause temporary nausea, especially in neurovegetative overload (e.g., overwork, stress, long journeys). In rare cases, bile can irritate the empty intestines, which will convulsively contract and push the bile toward the stomach. The stomach will rid itself of the bile by vomiting. Once this has passed, the fasting person feels relieved and well. It is recommended that you rest, place heat on the abdomen, and drink small sips of tepid chamomile tea (only if you like chamomile tea). Beverages that you have a distaste for should be avoided.

To speed up the process, you can induce vomiting yourself by expeditiously drinking a large glass of water containing a little salt.

Heartburn, Flatulence

At the beginning of a fast, the unbuffered gastric juices may irritate the mucous membrane. Rest and relaxation slow down the acid production. Cooked barley, oatmeal, or wheat bran (1 or 2 teaspoons with a little water) buffer the acid and alleviate the problem. Fasting beverages should be limited to weak (warm, not too hot) herbal teas, for example, chamomile, and diluted juices, for example, grape or beetroot juice. Honey should be omitted.

Leg Cramps

During the first days of a fast, leg cramps are associated with changes in the mineral balance, especially in people that have taken diuretic medication or laxatives for an extended period. Potassium, magnesium, and calcium supplements or a pinch of salt in the vegetable broth may afford relief.

Heart Palpitations

Changes in the mineral and water balance, especially in the first days during the sympathetic phase, as well as vegetative changes may lead to heart palpitations. In this case, phytotherapy and mineral supplements are helpful. Cardiac diseases must be ruled out diagnostically.

Restless Legs

This annoying sensation of restlessness occurs usually at night when lying down. It can be ameliorated by hot–cold or cold calf affusions and drinking plenty of liquids.

Hunger Feelings

A fasting person usually does not feel hungry. The blood contains plenty of »food« mainly as fat molecules. The gas gauge shows full! True hunger, generally felt in the area of the stomach, may occur in people with sensitive stomachs and also if the intestines were not entirely emptied. The hunger feeling is more often experienced by skinny individuals. Colon hydrotherapy or taking Epsom salts and colon massage are recommended. Hunger may permanently persist if the fast is subconsciously rejected (e.g., out of fear).

Food Cravings

If no signs of true hunger are present, for example, unpleasant sensation of emptiness in the stomach, and yet an enormous desire to eat is experienced, emotional issues are usually the underlying condition. The craving can be induced by minor stimulants, such as scents, images, or the window of a pastry shop. Suddenly there is the desire for certain foods (e.g., chocolate, salad, crunchy bread, aromatic cheese, or a juicy steak).

If this urge is brought to consciousness in a therapeutic setting, the craving usually subsides. If this craving cannot be remedied but is only suppressed, it may result in binge-eating that leads to the termination of the fast. Should this occur, the building-up phase is started and possible feelings of guilt and lowered self-esteem must be treated with the aid of psychotherapy.

Temporary Visual Impairment

During the fast, visual functions may be impaired while reading. Do not change your reading glasses, because the visual functions will return to the pre-fasting condition. This temporary visual impairment is associated with decreased intraocular pressure, which causes an alteration in the base curve of the lens. In cases of glaucoma, the decrease of intraocular pressure has beneficial effects.

Halitosis

Bad breath may be the result of ketosis, paradontosis (inflammation of the gums), or gases that have developed in the intestines and are now exhaled. In any case, brush your teeth and your tongue and watch your oral hygiene.

Dry Mouth

A dry mouth is most likely the consequence of the change in mineral balance, especially potassium balance, which reduces saliva production. Drink plenty of liquids, use lip balm, and add mineral supplements if necessary.

Skin Rash

A skin rash can be combined with itching; it may appear in a specific area or, less frequently, on the entire body. It can also appear at any time in the course of the fast and is considered a symptom of elimination. Either the skin is irritated by the acidic products of elimination dissolved in sweat or allergens or other substances (e.g., medication) that have been stored in the adipose tissue and now trigger an allergic reaction. It is recommended to take bran baths, stimulate the elimination via kidneys, intestines, and lungs, and take some alkaline powder.

Hypoglycemia

People who fast are energetic and are able to be active for many hours, but they should avoid maximum performance, which requires sugar for fueling. If you overexert yourself you risk a hypoglycemic attack, which ultimately leads to fatigue and sore muscles. Remedy: rest and drink tea with a bit of honey.

Changes in the Quality of Sleep

It is a frequent occurrence that people sleep for shorter periods when fasting but the sleep is equally refreshing. There is no need to force oneself

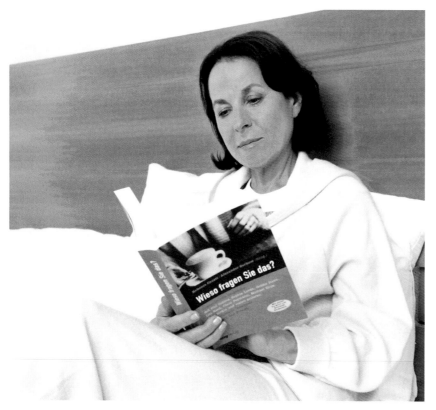

to sleep longer. Simply get up, refresh yourself with an early morning walk, pray, write, read, or spend your time on body care. Should you wake up during the night, just take it easy. When you fast you do not have to work the next day or make any kind of effort. You may as well use your midday break to catch up with sleep. The changes in sleeping patterns are associated either with hormonal changes at the beginning of a fast, including an elevated adrenaline level, or with mental–emotional issues and conflicts that manifest themselves in dreams, which wake you up. Solution: allow these thoughts and emotions, remember dreams and write them down; in cases of anxiety, say a prayer if this is an option for you, or get up, go outside, and inhale some fresh air.

》 Dr. Otto Buchinger recommended to people who had problems sleeping during their fast that they should not take sleeping pills but take the opportunity to learn a psalm or poem by heart! He said that ›a sleepless night can sometimes be a blessing.‹«

Weight Stagnation

Generally, weight stagnation happens when the body retains salt (sodium) and water; this is frequently observed in people who take diuretic medication or drink mineral water with a high sodium content before fasting. Sometimes a paradoxical reaction is possible. When sweating a lot due to physical exercise or extensive sauna sessions, large amounts of minerals are exuded as well. As a result, the body retains minerals and water and weight stagnates instead of being reduced.

In women, the reason for weight stagnation can be premenstrual water retention. Keep calm, the daily fat reduction still takes place, even if the scale does not indicate it. In rare cases, weight stagnation may be a sign of hypothyroidism.

Mood Disorders

These include depression, anxiety, and sadness; even if fasting has the tendency to improve the mood, de-pressed periods may arise and are usually considered an »initial aggravation.« Suppressed conflicts, unconscious shortcomings, and grief work their way into consciousness. You can come to terms with these issues with the help of a psychotherapist.

Attack of Gout

Especially in the beginning of a fasting period, the fat metabolism slows down the elimination of uric acid via the kidneys. This may cause the uric acid level to rise. If you do not drink enough or had elevated uric acid levels prior to the fast, an attack of gout (acute inflammation of the joint) may result. This can be remedied through the prescription of proper medication, if necessary.

- Onset of an infectious disease
- Spasmodic episode in porphyria
- Acute complaints in areas of scars
- Exacerbation of a pre-existing condition

Risks of Drug Therapies

Great caution must be exercised when the following medications are taken:
- Non-steroidal anti-rheumatic agents (NSAR)
- Systemic corticosteroids (max. 20 mg/day prednisone or equivalent)
- Antihypertensives (especially beta-blockers, diuretics)
- Anti-diabetics and insulin
- Contraceptives (limited effect)
- Anticoagulants (e.g., warfarin, Plavix (clopidogrel)
- Psychotropic drugs (especially neuroleptics and lithium)
- Anti-epileptics

Drug therapies must be under medical supervision. It is a challenge for the physician in charge of the fasting person to properly deal with a person's already existing drug therapy.

Fasting Crises

When fasting in a good place, away from everyday life, with proper medical care, fasting crises are the exception, even during extended fasts. A statistic compiled in our clinic shows that in the course of 3 months, only one of 350 patients suffered cardiac arrhythmia on the 17th day of the fast. He was released from hospital after 24 hours and successfully completed the fast.

People of good physical and psychological health run very little risk of experiencing a fasting crisis when they fast for 1 week. Nevertheless, it should not be ruled out completely, which is one reason we recommend having a physician on the sidelines.

The symptoms indicating a fasting crisis include the following:
- Migraine
- Incessant vomiting
- Ketoacidosis
- Biliary, renal, or intestinal colic
- Cardiac disorders, cardiac arrhythmia

The Buchinger Amplius Clinics in Überlingen and Marbella

In Germany, the Buchinger-Wilhelmi group is renowned for its clinics and its methods. In 1986, their efforts to develop a scientific base for fasting therapies, especially the impetus injected by Dr. Fahrner and Dr. Lützner, led to the foundation of the »Ärztegesellschaft Heilfasten und Ernährung« (ÄGHE; Medical Society for Fasting and Nutrition). In 2002, a group of experts consented to and published the *Guidelines for Therapeutic Fasting*.

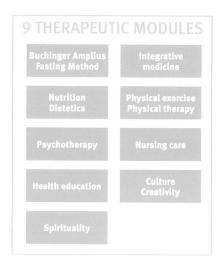

9 THERAPEUTIC MODULES

Buchinger Amplius Fasting Method	Integrative medicine
Nutrition Dietetics	Physical exercise Physical therapy
Psychotherapy	Nursing care
Health education	Culture Creativity
Spirituality	

The task of the physician specializing in fasting is to transform the fasting person into the subject of the process, motivate him/her, and support his/her autonomy. The physician listens actively and with empathy and encourages the individual. This allows a person to take an active part in his/her healing. The table on the right outlines five of the nine modules that are listed in the figure. They are modules that are part of every decent rehabilitation concept, including integrative medicine, nutrition and diet, physical therapy and physical exercise, psychotherapy, and nursing care. These five building blocks are employed in different set-ups, depending on the individual condition.

▲ The nine-module program, »Buchinger Amplius,« developed from the medically supervised, multidisciplinary therapeutic in-patient fasting concept at the Buchinger Amplius clinic in Überlingen, Germany.

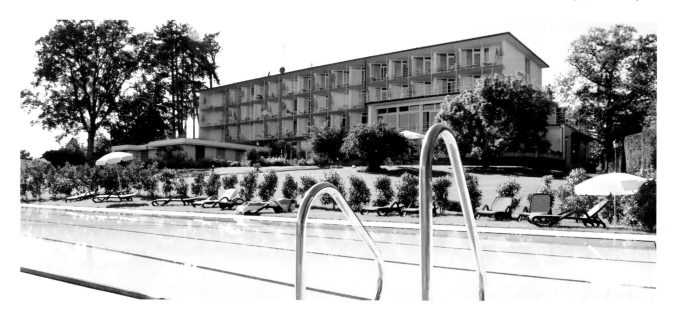

Five of the nine therapeutic modules of the Buchinger Amplius fasting program

Integrative medicine	Nutrition/ dietetics	Physical therapy/ exercise	Psychotherapy	Nursing care
▪ Holistic care and compilation of individual adaptation of the fasting programs ▪ Internal medicine: diagnosis and therapy ▪ Traditional European medicine (e.g., Kneipp hydrotherapy, homeopathy) and from other cultural spheres (e.g., TCM and ayurveda) ▪ Phytotherapy ▪ Aromatherapy ▪ Roeder method ▪ Autogenic training ▪ Lectures	▪ Fasting and building-up nutrition ▪ Organic whole foods, also low-calorie ▪ Training kitchen ▪ Training buffets ▪ Lectures ▪ Dietary counseling ▪ Cooking lessons	▪ Partial and full body massages ▪ Several treatments of naturopathy (e.g., reflexology, osteopathy, colonics, hydrotherapy and Kneipp therapy ▪ Applications from other cultural spheres (e.g., shiatsu, tuina, tai chi, qi gong, yoga) ▪ Therapeutic exercises ▪ Personal training ▪ Hiking ▪ Gymnastics	▪ Talking therapy ▪ Behavioral therapy emphasizing eating patterns ▪ Guided imagery ▪ Professional coaching ▪ Partner therapy ▪ Deep psychological counseling ▪ Dream work ▪ Art therapy ▪ Breathing therapy ▪ (Individual and group therapy)	▪ Daily care of fasting guests ▪ Emotional support ▪ Hot-liver pack ▪ Intestinal hygiene

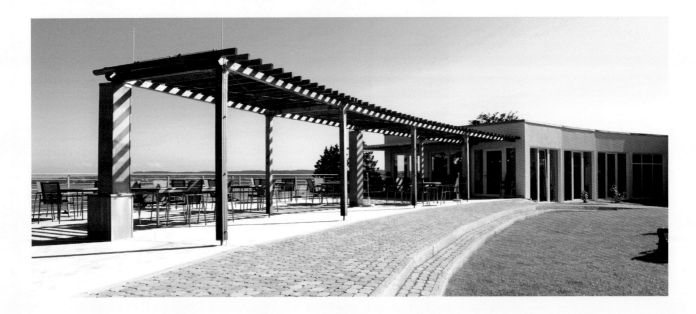

Let's Get Started: Suggestions and Tips for Your Fast

Take as much time as you can for the transition from hectic everyday life, work, or whatever the stressors in your life may be, into your fasting period. The emblematic jump-in at the deep end is not recommended.

We do not suggest that you begin your fast with »the last meal.« We would rather like to encourage you to reduce coffee and alcohol consumption, maybe even eliminate it, and eat less meat and more fresh products. This makes for a smoother transition into the fast. We do realize that many people fast because they view it as their lifebuoy as too many areas of their lives are out of control, for example, excessive food, excessive work, not enough sleep, and not enough joy. Whatever the reason or the approach, before starting a fast, at least 1 day of transition is necessary.

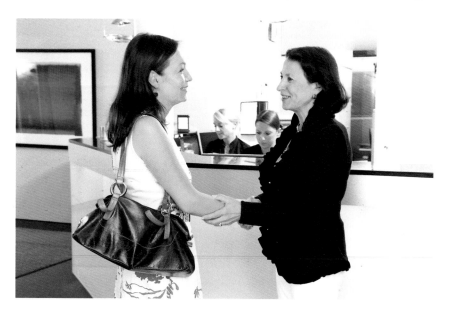

If you fast in a clinic, the transition day should follow the arrival day. In the case of a short fast, arrival and pre-cleansing day can be the same. And please, I urge you not to omit the building-up days after the fast. Those are the most critical days, especially if you want to maintain your weight loss.

In the section below, I will provide you with suggestions and information on how to organize:

- the arrival day, in case you fast in a clinic;
- the transition day;
- the actual fasting period;
- breaking the fast;
- returning to a regular diet (building-up days).

On pages 98–99 you will find a table listing our suggestions for a 10-day fast (1 transition day, 5 actual fasting days, 1 day breaking the fast, and 3 building-up days).

your first time fasting, make the day after your arrival your transition day.

Allow yourself a gentle transition into your fast, particularly if you have no experience in fasting or if you feel truly exhausted, physically or mentally! Do not think of it as a loss of your »real« fasting period. Your metabolism will be grateful!

Menu for the Body
A light meal without alcohol, coffee, and meat; or the transition day with mono-diet (rice, fruit, potatoes, or oats divided into three to four meals, see pp. 110–114).

Menu for the Soul
Stress-free arrival. Be aware of the racing and the overabundance of your thoughts.

Motto of the Day
Take your time to unpack, make yourself at home in your guestroom, and »arrive.«

Arrival Day When You Fast in a Clinic

» The Buchinger tradition places great value on a smooth and calm metabolic transition into fasting. The arrival day is often characterized by a change of place, time, climate, and sometimes even language. Therefore, if this is

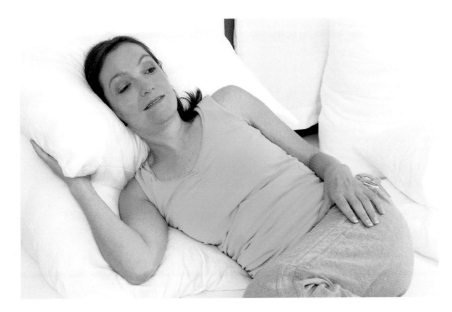

» Alcohol, tobacco, and junk food keep preparing the soil for our medical waiting room harvest.«
Otto Buchinger

◀ On the arrival day, take your time to get settled and familiarize yourself with your new surroundings.

Transition Day

» Consciously attune yourself to your upcoming fast on the transition day.

Menu for the Body
Eating and Drinking
- Drink plenty of water and herbal tea.
- Mono-diet (rice, fruit, potatoes, or oats divided into three to four meals; see pp. 110–114).

Detox
- The large cellulose portion of the mono-diet and large amounts of liquids produce soft colon contents.
- Get plenty of rest.

Exercising
- Go for walks, as desired.

Care and Hygiene
- Come to rest.
- Take a bath if you feel like it.

Menu for the Soul
- Say farewell to everyday life, your fasting period is free of obligations.
- Allow yourself as much rest as you need.
- Prepare yourself mentally for the fasting days to come, maybe you would like to make a note of something.
- Pay attention to your needs and your body language.
- Pay attention to your dreams and have pen and paper ready.

» Instead of asking yourself: ›What have I lost?,‹ always ask yourself: ›What is left?‹«

Otto Buchinger

First Fasting Day (Cleansing Day)

» The time has come. You do not ingest solid foods any longer. This enables your body to switch to the nutritional program II, the internal nutrition from fat reserves.

Menu for the Body
Eating and Drinking
Drink water and herbal teas, ca. 2 to 3 L with 1 to 2 teaspoons of honey in the course of the day.
- Early: morning tea and Glauber's salt (see p. 72).
- Mid-morning: drink plenty of liquids (water or tea ca. 1 hour after taking the Glauber's salt).
- Midday: 250 mL freshly squeezed fruit or vegetable juice (also organic grade bottled juice).
- Evening: 250 mL vegetable broth.

Detox
- Mid-morning, thorough emptying of the bowels via Glauber's salt (or colonic irrigation).
- Stay within easy reach of a bathroom for a few hours.
- Hot liver pack following the fasting beverage at midday (1 to 2 hours).

Exercising
- Morning exercise after bowel movements.
- Otherwise, rest, do some yoga exercises, if you wish to, and have a colon massage.

Care and Hygiene
- Take a bath and/or do some dry brushing when you feel like it.
- Treat possible bad breath by cleaning your tongue, brushing your teeth, and having a mouthwash (one drop of peppermint oil diluted in water).
- Go to bed early at night.

Second Fasting Day

Menu for the Soul
- Become aware of your body; what do you need right now?
- Consciously observe the slow disappearance of the hunger feeling. Visualize how the body switches to internal nutrition and the digestive tract is cleansed. Trustingly accept the changes. Discomforts that may present themselves are usually reactions to the adaptation; if the reactions disconcert you, speak to a physician or the fasting counselor about them.
- Pay attention to your moods.
- Be good to yourself and satisfy your needs if possible.

》 Wealth may only claim a right to exist due to culture and charity.«

Otto Buchinger

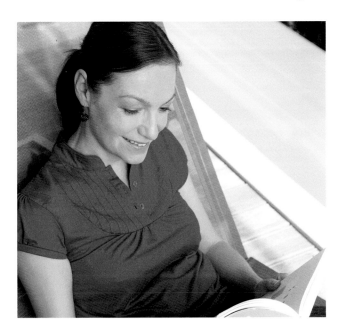

》 Give yourself permission to be active or passive, depending on your momentary needs. The physical hunger subsides, but what does your soul need?

Menu for the Body
Eating and Drinking
Drink water and herbal teas, ca. 2 to 3 L with 1 to 2 teaspoons of honey in the course of the day.
- Early: morning tea (possibly with honey).
- Midday: 250 mL freshly squeezed fruit or vegetable juice (also organic grade bottled juice).
- Evening: 250 mL vegetable broth.

Detox
- Drink large amounts of water until the color of urine is very light.
- Exercise deep respiration (see pp. 66–69).

Starting the Exercise Program
- Stretching and gymnastics or yoga.
- Go for a 1- to 2-hour walk or hike (pace: you can breathe through the nose without effort).

Care and Hygiene
- Hot liver pack following the fasting beverage at midday (1 to 2 hours).
- Apply organic grade oil or lotion to your entire body.
- Get a massage or another treatment if you like.

Menu for the Soul
- Allow yourself to stay in bed longer if you feel like it. Do you need solitude and quiet or the stimulation of a conversation and some company?
- Still, consider any discomfort a symptom of the adaptation; it generally passes! You are obliged to nothing and nobody.
- Write in your diary!

Third Fasting Day

» This is usually the day when the energy during the fast stabilizes.

Menu for the Body

Eating and Drinking

Drink water and herbal teas, ca. 2 to 3 L with 1 to 2 teaspoons of honey in the course of the day.

- Early: morning tea (possibly with honey).
- Midday: 250 mL freshly squeezed fruit or vegetable juice (also organic grade bottled juice).
- Evening: 250 mL vegetable broth.

Detox

- Induce bowel movement via colonic irrigation and follow with a colon massage (if necessary use Epsom salts instead).
- Make sure your urine is of light color.

Intensifying the Exercise Program

- Extend your stretching and gymnastics or yoga.
- Extend your walk/hike (pace: you can breathe through the nose without effort).

Care and Hygiene

- Hot liver pack following the fasting beverage at midday (1 to 2 hours).
- Give yourself a dry brushing massage followed by a shower, and oil/lotion application.

Menu for the Soul

- You most likely have cleared the hurdle of adaptation by now. Enjoy the new energy! You can applaud yourself a little, if you have remained confident.
- Otherwise: take your time, enjoy nature, listen to music, read, write, talk, or do whatever makes you happy.
- Realize consciously how your body has adapted to the fasting metabolism.
- Make sure that you maintain your body temperature by dressing properly, exercising, drinking warm beverages, utilizing the hot-water bottle, and having a sauna, as appropriate.
- Ask for your dreams and listen to your inner voice!

» Dedicate at least half an hour a day to reflection on the meaning of your life; ultimately, your achievements will thrive.«

Otto Buchinger

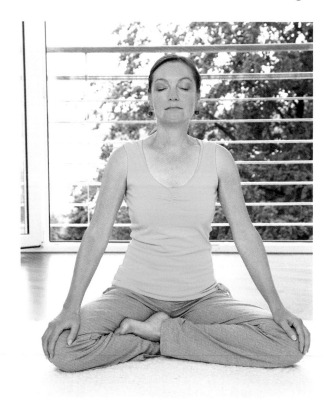

Additional Fasting Days

Take stock of your life. Consciously experience the joys and ease of life while you are on »autopilot.« If it is helpful, seek supportive talks (also of pastoral or psychotherapeutic nature).

Menu for the Body

Eating and Drinking

Drink water and herbal teas, ca. 2 to 3 L with 1 to 2 teaspoons of honey in the course of the day.
- Early: morning tea (possibly with honey).
- Midday: 250 mL freshly squeezed fruit or vegetable juice (also organic grade bottled juice).
- Evening: 250 mL vegetable broth.

Detox
- Have colonic irrigation every other day, followed by a colon massage.

Intensifying the Exercise Program
- Extend your stretching and gymnastics or yoga.
- Extend your walk/hike (pace: you can breathe through the nose without effort).

Care and Hygiene
- Hot liver pack following the fasting beverage at midday (1 to 2 hours).
- Give yourself a dry brushing massage followed by a shower, and oil/lotion application.

Menu for the Soul
- Have positive thoughts about your loved ones as well as people you are in conflict with. Write a letter or make a phone call.
- Try to remain silent for half a day or the entire day.

FROM MY EXPERIENCES

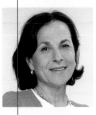

Detoxification—Spiritual Cleansing

During a fast, physical or spiritual cleansing may occur. All the conflicts, problems, or questions that currently occupy your mind may become more evident and obvious, because the everyday distractions are missing. The fast offers a time to take a look at your own life.

Keep a diary and use the time to face up to any issue that presents itself. If a problem or a conflict, for example, with my partner or family, occupies my mind, I ask myself what do I wish for? What would I like to achieve? I consider my options. If I cannot find a solution, in spite of my best efforts, I try to let go of it. I tell myself that I do not have a solution at this moment and ask for a dream, a sign, or an encounter to indicate the next step. The wish is passed on to intuition. Whenever I have been clear about my wish and was able to formulate it that way, something along these lines has taken place.

》 Every challenge that comes your way exists so you can prove yourself and master it, not to defeat you.«

Otto Buchinger

Breaking the Fast

» How are you? Would you like to continue fasting or are you looking forward to eating again?

Menu for the Body

Eating and Drinking

Drink water and herbal teas, ca. 2 to 3 L with 1 to 2 teaspoons of honey in the course of the day.
- Early: morning tea (possibly with honey).
- Mid-morning: an apple or a small bowl of stewed apples and two filberts or cashews.
- Midday: 250 mL vegetable broth or 250 mL freshly squeezed fruit or vegetable juice.
- Afternoon: an apple or a small bowl of stewed apples and two filberts or cashews.
- Evening: carrot and potato soup (see recipe p. 115).

Detox
- Make sure your urine is of light color.
- Hot liver pack following the fasting beverage at midday (1 to 2 hours).

Maintaining the Exercise Program
- Stretching and gymnastics or yoga.
- Daily walks or hikes.
- Listen to your body.
- Food shopping for the building-up phase.

Menu for the Soul
- Have supportive talks (also of pastoral or psychotherapeutic nature) if you feel that your life requires some changes.
- Do not view your fast as being completed, only after the building-up phase.
- Celebrate your meals and enjoy the delicate sense of taste. Enjoy the return of your regular body heat.
- Pay attention to hunger and satiety.

» Appease your hunger and keep your appetite.«
Otto Buchinger

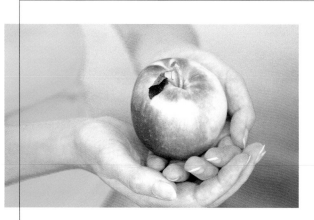

KNOWLEDGE

The Apple Ritual
- Enjoy eating your first apple.
- Eat slowly and chew it well.
- Only eat until you have had enough. It could be that you cannot eat the whole apple.
- The apple is more easily digestible if you cut it into small pieces and sauté it briefly.
- In addition, you may eat four nuts.

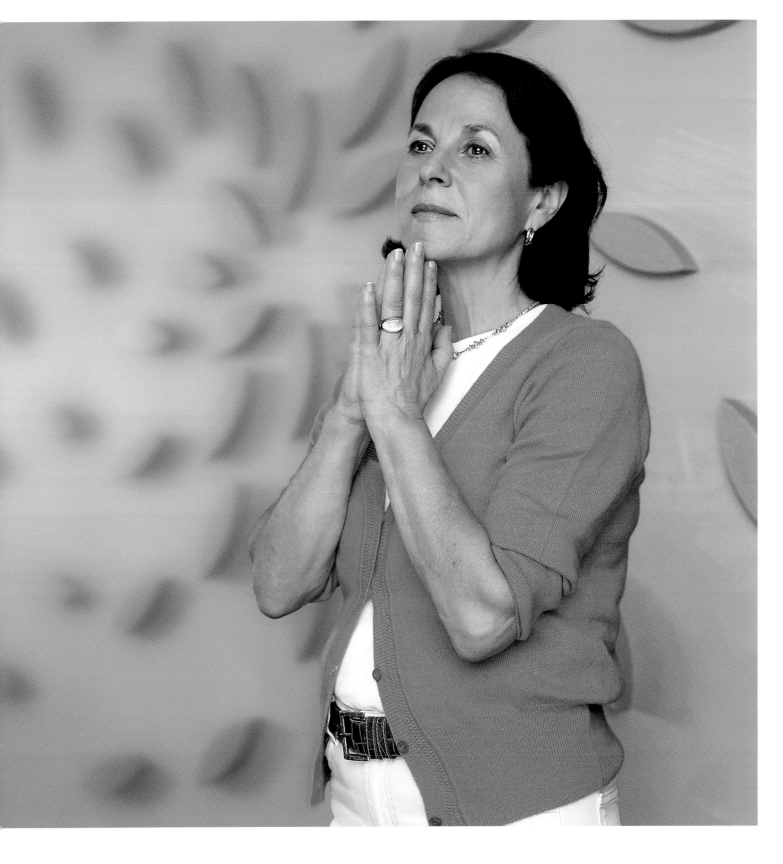

An outline for your 10-day fasting program

	Arrival day*	Day 1 Pre-cleansing day	Day 2 First fasting day	Day 3 Second fasting day	Day 4 Third fasting day	
Motto of the day	Getting comfortable with the surroundings	Deceleration and metabolic adaptation	Letting go and elimination	Realizing and attending to one's needs	Energetic release	
Early	▪ Light vegetarian breakfast, e.g., muesli	▪ Mono-diet (rice, fruit, potatoes, or oats), see pp. 110–114	▪ Drink the correct quantity of Glauber's salt solution for your individual requirements	▪ Herbal tea	▪ Herbal tea	
Mid-morning	▪ Drink plenty of water and tea	▪ Drink plenty of water and tea ▪ Take time for yourself	▪ Drink plenty of water and herbal tea ▪ Take time for yourself ▪ Stay at home	▪ Drink plenty of water and herbal tea ▪ Take time for yourself	▪ Drink plenty of water and herbal tea ▪ Colonic irrigation ▪ Take time for yourself	
Midday	▪ Light vegetarian meal	▪ Mono-diet (rice, fruit, potatoes, or oats) ▪ Midday nap with hot liver pack	▪ 250 mL fruit or vegetable juice ▪ Midday nap with hot liver pack	▪ 250 mL fruit or vegetable juice ▪ Midday nap with hot liver pack	▪ 250 mL fruit or vegetable juice ▪ Midday nap with hot liver pack	
Afternoon	▪ Siesta, arrival, getting comfortable with the new surroundings, arranging everything for one's needs	▪ Drink plenty of water and tea ▪ Go for a hike or a walk	▪ Drink herbal tea with honey and/or lemon ▪ Go for a hike or a walk	▪ Drink herbal tea with honey and/or lemon ▪ Go for a hike or a walk	▪ Drink herbal tea with honey and/or lemon ▪ Go for a hike or a walk	
Evening	▪ Light vegetarian meal	▪ Mono-diet (rice, fruit, potatoes, or oats)	▪ 250 mL vegetable broth	▪ 250 mL vegetable broth	▪ 250 mL vegetable broth	
Caloric intake		ca. 600–800 kcal	ca. 250 kcal	ca. 250 kcal	ca. 250 kcal	

* In case you do not fast at home.

Day 5 Fourth fasting day	Day 6 Fifth fasting day	Day 7 Breaking the fast	Day 8 First building-up day	Day 9 Second building-up day	Day 10 Third building-up day
Desire for movement Adjustment ensues	Hunger has vanished Satisfaction, absence of need Cheerfulness	One eye laughing, the other eye weeping	Hunger and satiety return and control food intake	Remain cautious: your eyes are bigger than your stomach	The big caterpillar turns into a butterfly
▪ Drink herbal tea	▪ Drink herbal tea	▪ Drink herbal tea	▪ Herbal tea and quinoa apple puree (recipe see p. 116)	▪ Herbal tea, Budwig cream with fruit (recipe see p. 120)	▪ Herbal tea, Budwig cream with fruit (recipe see p. 120)
▪ Drink plenty of water and herbal tea ▪ Take time for yourself	▪ Drink plenty of water and herbal tea ▪ Colonic irrigation ▪ Take time for yourself	▪ Drink plenty of water ▪ Colonic irrigation, if necessary ▪ Shopping for the rebuilding phase	▪ Take time for yourself	▪ Take time for yourself	▪ Take time for yourself
▪ 250 mL fruit or vegetable juice ▪ Midday nap with hot liver pack	▪ 250 mL fruit or vegetable juice ▪ Midday nap with hot liver pack	▪ One apple (raw or stewed) to be savored to the full ▪ Midday nap with hot liver pack	▪ Belgian endive salad, mashed potatoes with spinach (recipe see p. 116) ▪ Midday nap with hot liver pack	▪ Green salad, quinoa soufflé (recipe see p. 120) ▪ Midday nap with hot liver pack	▪ Sauerkraut salad, Belgian endive with bulgur (recipe see p. 124) ▪ Midday nap with hot liver pack
▪ Drink herbal tea with honey and/or lemon ▪ Go for a hike or a walk	▪ Drink herbal tea with honey and/or lemon ▪ Go for a hike or a walk	▪ Fruit, herbal tea with honey and lemon ▪ Continue drinking plenty of water ▪ Go for a hike or a walk	▪ Fruit, herbal tea with honey and lemon ▪ Continue drinking plenty of water ▪ Go for a hike or a walk	▪ Fruit, herbal tea with honey and lemon ▪ Continue drinking plenty of water ▪ Go for a hike or a walk	▪ Fruit, herbal tea with honey and lemon ▪ Continue drinking plenty of water ▪ Go for a hike or a walk
▪ 250 mL vegetable broth	▪ 250 mL vegetable broth	▪ Carrot and potato soup (recipe see p. 115)	▪ Fennel, vegetable potpourri with rice (recipe see p. 118)	▪ Zucchini salad, potatoes with Budwig cream and beetroot (recipe see p. 122)	▪ Celery, vegetable millet soufflé (recipe see p. 124)
ca. 250 kcal	ca. 250 kcal	ca. 350 kcal	800 kcal	1000 kcal	1200 kcal

Deliberately Designing the Building-up Phase

Breaking the fast and returning to a regular diet correspond to the »landing« phase. Enjoy the building-up phase, but remain cautious! The lasting effects of the fast depend on a successful building-up phase! From the moment of breaking the fast, the fasting metabolism slowly returns to the eating mode by default.

Allow yourself 3 building-up days (after fasting for 5 days). If the purpose of your fast was weight reduction, the building-up phase is crucial! You are on the right track if you manage to change your nutrition in the way that we outline for you.

What Happens During the Building-up Phase?

» The first bite into an apple awakens the gastrointestinal tract. The digestive processes start up to supply the body with fuel and building blocks obtained from food.

Eat slowly and chew the food thoroughly. This stimulates the production of saliva and digestive juices, facilitates the work of the digestive organs, and allows you to fully enjoy the flavors that you had to do without for a while.

Every digestive tract re-starts at a different pace, therefore, watch your physical signs: flatulence, abdominal discomfort, and a feeling of heaviness in the stomach should be avoided. Stay calm, even if the return of bowel movements takes until the fourth building-up day! For spontaneous elimination to occur, the colon has to fill all the way to the rectum. Colonic irrigation can help if nothing happens on the fifth building-up day. Some wheat bran mixed with an ample amount of liquids may be helpful if constipation was already present before the fast. Exercise, colon massage, and the absence of stress are also beneficial during the building-up phase. During the first hours of the building-up phase, fatigue may be experienced in place of the expected surge of energy. This is caused by the

KNOWLEDGE

The Challenge of the Building-up Phase

On the one hand, the body's reserves have to be replenished and some proteic structures must be rebuilt. On the other hand, it takes a few days until digestion functions completely. This is a challenge to the body. The art of building up the diet lies in ingesting foods of ideal quality (as natural as possible) and yet to avoid flatulence, a feeling of fullness, or abdominal discomfort.

People who were able to eat everything without experiencing digestive problems prior to the fast, usually encounter fewer difficulties during the building-up phase. People whose digestion is weak may find the building-up phase trying. They should eat slowly, chew thoroughly, eat less raw foods, have small simple meals, and support their digestion through heat applications, exercise, and abdominal treatments.

increased perfusion of the digestive tract, which in turn requires a change in blood distribution. Be patient! Rest after meals, walks, and composure will help the regained vitality to flood the entire body shortly.

The term »building-up« indicates that the vitamin, glycogen, and, in normal-weight people, fat storages, have to be replenished. Simultaneously, some protein structures are quickly rebuilt, for example, on the intestinal surface,

digestive enzymes, or muscular proteins. Whole foods that are individually agreeable must be used during the building-up phase. Nutrition during the building-up phase is light and lacto-ovo vegetarian; it contains whole foods, and unsaturated fats (cold-pressed vegetable oils containing omega 3 and 6 in the cis-cis form). The first building-up day provides ca. 800 kcal, the second ca. 1000 kcal, and the third ca. 1200 kcal. You should continue drinking plenty between meals.

miss the lightness of being on autopilot and the serotonin-induced harmonization of emotions. After eating the first apple, some feel like Adam and Eve banished from the peaceful existence in paradise!

》 The sated, fat caterpillar pupates. Motionless, in its chitin coffin, the seemingly dead creature fasts for 6 to 7 months, until the warm spring sun bursts its cocoon. It is not the same shapeless ugly caterpillar that exits, but an unfolded, buoyant creature, a butterfly. It is not without good reason that it has always been the symbol of our soul.«

Otto Buchinger

The time has come to say goodbye to the fast, the »fasting cell,« the support team, the fasting group that one has grown fond of, and the security; to spread one's wings again, and to return to everyday life.

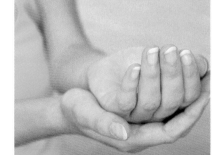

Returning to Everyday Life

》 People who are experienced in fasting report that they face the building-up phase with one eye laughing and one eye weeping. They enjoy the return-

ing warmth, the renewed energy, and the restored ability to relish nutrition, which turns simple meals into a feast for the senses. At the same time, they

First Building-up Day

» Just like the first fasting day, the first building-up day is a day for adjustment, which may be accompanied by fatigue or any type of disorder.

Menu for the Body

Eating and Drinking

Continue to drink plenty of water or tea.

- Early: morning tea, oat or spelt porridge with stewed fruit.
- Midday: small raw foods dish, potatoes in the skin with curd and flax seed oil, steamed vegetables.
- Evening: millet, steamed vegetables with sunflower oil.

Detox

- Midday nap, heat application on the abdomen.
- Fill the intestines slowly and carefully, chew thoroughly.

Exercise

Continue your exercise program just like you did while fasting; adjust it to your change in performance.

Care and Hygiene

Hot liver or stomach compress (move the compress from the liver area to the stomach area) during the midday rest (rest for at least 1 hour).

▶ Raw foods are sometimes hard to digest. Pay attention to their individual palatability.

Menu for the Soul

- Consciously experience the ambivalence of the situation: on the one hand it is great to eat again, to feel the energy and warmth return to the body.
- On the other hand it is sad to feel the loss of serenity and cheerfulness that was present during the fast.
- Deliberately enjoy eating, but practice moderation as well. Only eat when you are truly hungry! Chew thoroughly and speak as little as possible during a meal. The intake of water into the digestive tract and the general tissues can produce an increase in weight of up to 1 kg, despite continuous fat reduction.

» You cannot give more than yourself. But you must not give less than that.«

Otto Buchinger

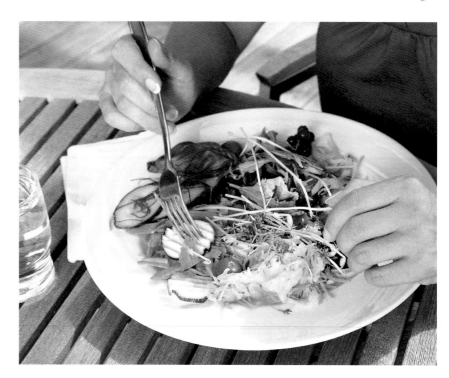

Additional Building-up Days

» The building-up phase following a therapeutic fast frequently depends on the indication. Fewer foods may be advantageous, for example, omitting dairy products, gluten, meats, and animal products.

Menu for the Body

Eating and Drinking

Increase the amounts of food slowly and carefully and continue to drink plenty of water.

- Early: morning tea, Budwig cream by Dr. Kousmine (if you can tolerate it; see recipe, p. 120), otherwise oat or spelt porridge with stewed fruit.
- Midday: raw foods dish, or freshly squeezed juice, or vegetable soup with sunflower oil, whole grains (e.g., rice) or potatoes, steamed vegetables with cold-pressed sunflower oil, vinegar, and herbs.
- Protein components: dairy products (cheese or curd), legumes, or egg.
- After the fourth building-up day, you may add 100 g of fish or meat.
- Evening: menu following the same principle as lunch but without protein addition.

Detox

- Drink plenty of liquid and wait for spontaneous bowel movements to return around the third or fourth day of the building-up phase. It usually takes a few days until the intestines are sufficiently filled.

- You may help the body with a colon massage, physical activities, and dietary fiber (e.g., wheat bran).

Exercise

Continue your exercise program just like you did while fasting; adjust it to your change in performance but avoid overexertion.

Care and Hygiene

- Apply a hot liver or stomach compress during the midday rest (for at least 1 hour).

- In the morning, stimulate your circulatory system with dry brushing.

Menu for the Soul

- Prepare for your return to everyday life and finish your fasting diary.
- Think about how to enliven your everyday life, change your dietary habits, and set aside more time for yourself. Set yourself small but attainable goals (see box below) that you can realize in your everyday life.

» For the poor. Certainly. But who cares for the rich? They are usually in greater distress.«

Otto Buchinger

FROM MY EXPERIENCES

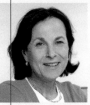

Introducing Changes into Everyday Life

Which realizations and experiences would you like to incorporate into your everyday life? Make concrete plans but be realistic about them. From my own experience, I know that fasting is an exceptional time, in which lofty plans are made. Back in everyday life, these plans are quickly dropped. Scale down your expectations to give yourself the chance to meet them. If you can realize small changes, your success will provide you with the motivation to continue making changes. You can, for example, plan to realize one positive change in each of the following areas: exercising, diet, and emotional well-being. After 1 week check if you were able to implement those changes and make adjustments as necessary.

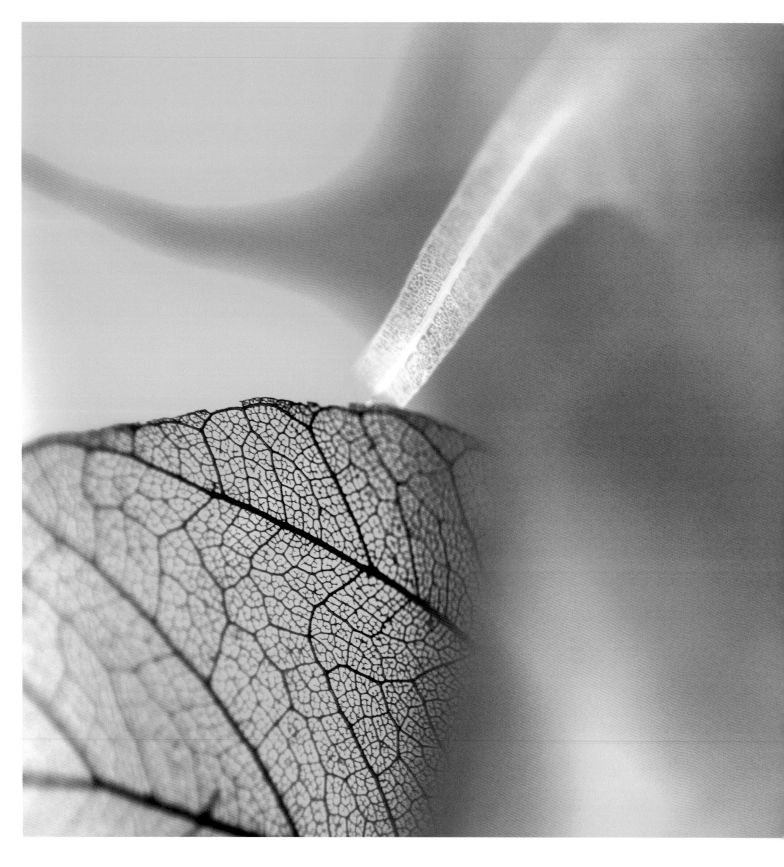

Eating Healthily after the Fast

During the fast, the digestive organs take a vacation. As a consequence, the intestinal mucous membrane diminishes and forms anew during the building-up phase. This is your chance for a new beginning and a change in eating habits. Together with the chef of our clinic, I will explain the significant aspects of this new beginning.

Enjoying Natural Foods

Consider eating after the fast a new beginning. Awareness and sensitivity to flavors have heightened. Hubert Hohler is the chef of our clinic. He fasts regularly and provides some suggestions for you.

Hubert Hohler: »The time following a fast is ideal to cultivate sensitivity toward natural flavors. Taste perception is newly sensitized through the break in eating.

Exploring the Sense of Taste

Explore the different taste sensations on your tongue. For example, dip a cotton swab into lemon juice and dab it on various areas of your tongue. Where does the lemon juice taste sour? What other qualities of taste do you notice? On what part of your tongue do you notice these qualities? Repeat the same with sweet, salty, or bitter liquids.

Now, let a spoonful of natural yoghurt melt on your tongue.

What do you taste? Try to discern the different qualities. Generally, a sour flavor is noticed first, including a slightly bitter flavor, which is followed by a sweet flavor caused by lactose.

Place a spoonful of yoghurt together with a slice of apple in your mouth next. Feel the different textures of the foods. What do you taste now? Does it taste sour or sweet? What do you notice first? What are the different apple aromas? Finally, add a piece of walnut. Chew and taste with relish. Take your time to perceive each individual taste sensation. The fats and different texture of the walnut intensify and prolong the taste experiences.«

Dr. Wilhelmi de Toledo: »You can enjoy simple and natural low-calorie foods, if you consciously perceive the abundance of taste sensations.«

Hubert Hohler: »This may be an acquired taste. If you have eaten primarily foods containing artificial aromas and flavor enhancers or intensely spiced or salted foods, you need to re-learn to perceive the taste of natural products.

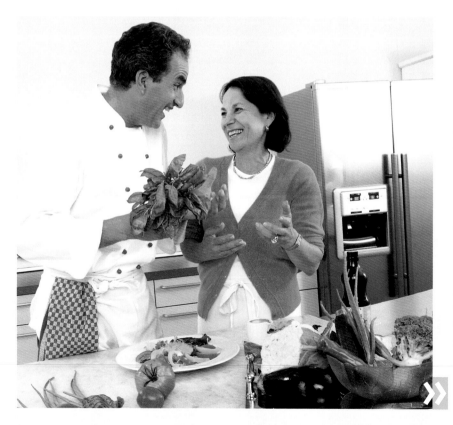

Use fresh, regional products that smell and look appetizing.

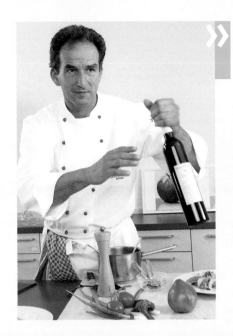

This can be easily done after a fast. After not eating anything for a while, you have weaned yourself off the old perceptions and have the opportunity to return to natural pleasures.

To me, yoghurt with artificial aromas seems to be way too crude; it lacks delicate stimulation.«

Dr. Wilhelmi de Toledo: »It is easy to reduce sugar and salt consumption after a fast. Mild stimulation is enough to produce enjoyment. There is no loss in pleasure; one has simply become more sensitive.

Fat is Not Generally a Bad Thing
There is a lot of confusion regarding the consumption and usefulness of fat. Let

When frying or sautéing, use as little fat as possible. Only when you reduce the heat should you add more high-quality oil.

us begin by talking about roasting and cooking.«

Hubert Hohler: »When using oil, the amount and quality of the oil are important and also the right timing. When you roast something with fat, you notice right away where the aromas go. They evaporate and are now in your hair and clothing but not in the food. This means, if you prepare food in a skillet or a pot, use oil initially as sparingly as possible. You can add more oil at the end when you do not need heat. At that time a small amount of oil suffices because the fat does not burn and the aroma remains within the food. I use high-quality, cold-pressed oil. You reduce fat, which means calories, but you do not diminish the enjoyment of eating. Try this for yourself.«

Dr. Wilhelmi de Toledo: »Olive oil is well suited up to 160°C. Special frying oils should be used if you need more heat.«

Hubert Hohler: »When I lightly sauté vegetables I use a small amount of olive oil. It contains primarily monounsaturated fatty acids and handles heat pretty well. The more polyunsaturated fatty acids oil contains, the lower the flash point. This means, at 120°C the oil begins to burn, harmful substances are

created, and the structures of the fatty acids change and form trans fatty acids. At the double bond, the oil is at its most sensitive toward heat and oxygen. The higher quality the oil is, for example, cold-pressed, the more unstable it is and more easily it turns rancid. Therefore, high-quality oils turn rancid easily. Flax seed oil contains many polyunsaturated omega-3 fatty acids and can be stored up to 3 months in the fridge. Olive oil contains primarily monounsaturated fatty acids and can be stored between 6 and 12 months. High-quality oil should be stored in a cool place, protected against light.«

Omega-6 and Omega-3 Fatty Acids
Dr. Wilhelmi de Toledo: »Most processed foods contain many harmful fats, such as hydrogenated fats. We usually also eat excessive amounts of the saturated fats, such as butter (milk fat). On the other hand, we do not eat enough essential fats. These are the polyunsaturated fatty acids in the form of either omega-6 or omega-3 fatty acids. Sunflower oil contains mainly omega-6 and flax seed oil mainly omega-3 fatty acids. Ideally, the ratio between omega-6 and omega-3 fatty acids should be 5:2. There is a plentiful omega-6 supply, unfortunately coming from low-grade sources (margarine). On the other hand, we usually do not eat enough omega-3 fatty acids because they are only found in a limited number of foods. Flax seed oil is a great vegetable source and fatty fish from cold waters, such as mackerel

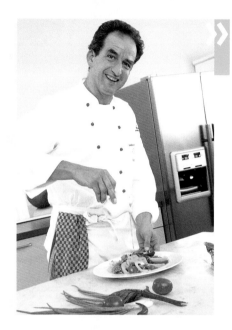

or salmon, is a great animal source of omega-3 fatty acids.«

Hubert Hohler: »Not to forget walnuts. Three walnuts a day cover one-quarter of our omega-3 fatty acid needs. The rule of thirds seems helpful to me in terms of fat intake. We should eat no more than 60 g of fat (600 kcal) per day:

- One-third should be polyunsaturated, including cold-pressed flax seed, canola, walnut, or sunflower oil (an example for the correct ratio: 1 tablespoon sunflower oil, 1 tablespoon flax seed oil).
- One-third should be monounsaturated (according to the ratio above: 2 tablespoons olive oil, for example to sauté vegetables).

Flax seed oil is a great vegetable source for omega-3 fatty acids. At the Buchinger clinic, it is a vital component of nutrition.

- One-third may be saturated (according to the ratio above: 20 g butter on the bread roll).«

Dr. Wilhelmi de Toledo: »Flax seed oil should be emulsified, which makes it more digestible. You can mix it with low-fat curd as part of your muesli, for example.«

Hubert Hohler: »Oil-bearing seeds must be chewed very well to be properly metabolized. In particular, flax seeds and sesame seeds will exit the body looking the way they did when they were eaten if they are simply swallowed. They must be soaked to macerate, minced, or crushed.«

Water Culture
Dr. Wilhelmi de Toledo: »One drinks a lot of water during the fast. This habit should be retained when the fast is over. We should cultivate our water consumption to cover our need for fluids and quench our thirst. Beverages that are recommended by advertisements often contain large amounts of sugar or alcohol. Our mixed drinks are, for example, based on tea (see recipe p. 152). Fruit juices are high-caloric beverages and should be watered down by one-half. The digestive organs had a break during the fast and must be

awakened slowly, otherwise indigestion will result. After the fast you have the opportunity to positively influence the reconstruction of the intestinal flora by eating whole foods and raw foods. How much of these foods are beneficial to you depends on your individual constitution.«

Hubert Hohler: »In terms of fasting, my focus as a chef is placed on the building-up phase rather than on fasting itself. The dietary habits change by shifting more toward crop products and vegetables and away from meats. You will be back in your initial state after approximately 1 month if you return to the same diet you had prior to the fast. Our motto is: eat slowly and deliberately and return to simple and natural foods! Make sure you shop for high-quality, basic foods.«

Sustainable Pleasure
Dr. Wilhelmi de Toledo: »Eat only when you are truly hungry. That is another vital principle. Even simple foods taste good when you are hungry. Choose regional, ecologically sound foods. What is healthy for humans is also good for the ecosystem of our planet.«

Hubert Hohler: »Sustainability plays an important role in my eyes. I cannot enjoy something if I know that others have to suffer because of it. Ethiopia, a famine-ridden country, is the second-largest food producer for European large-scale livestock farming. I do not

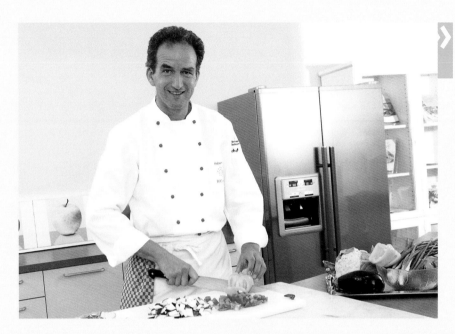

All fruits and vegetables are packed with vitamins. They are sensitive to heat and should therefore be eaten raw in proper amounts.

want to eat meat that is produced from that; it raises my hackles. My preferred nutrition stems from foods that grow naturally wherever it may be and do not give me the feeling that I take something away from someone else.«

Dr. Wilhelmi de Toledo: »Eating takes place not only in the mouth. Try to perceive foods with all your senses. It is probably much more enjoyable eating an apricot that is ripe, colorful, smells delightful, and tastes sweet and full of aromas than eating an apricot Danish where some orange-colored sugar pulp sticks to a pudding mass. I would love to eat the apricot but can do without the sugar-fat mixture. ›You become what you eat.‹«

Preserving Vitamins, Minerals, and Essential Fatty Acids

Hubert Hohler: »Food can be viewed as building blocks for the body. All vegetables that grow in the ground (soil) are mainly important as mineral sources. Minerals are dissolved in the soil and thereby absorbed by potatoes, carrots, or radishes. Minerals are thermo stable but water soluble, which means that they are washed out during the process of cooking. Little water should be used for cooking if the water is not further used for sauces or soups.

Meat quality depends on the animal feed. The omega-6/omega-3 imbalance in industrialized countries is partly due to the fact that cattle and poultry are fed with corn and soy instead of feeding

on green pastures. The preparation of whole foods does not have to be difficult. If at all possible, shop for organic, ripe products, because they contain better-developed secondary plant compounds and taste more intense. Proper storage is also important. Tomatoes, zucchini, and cucumbers do not like the cold of the refrigerator. Ideally, they are stored only for a brief time at approximately 13°C. Root vegetables are less sensitive and can be stored for longer periods of time. Carrots, beetroot, and cabbages can be refrigerated. If you consider the shelf-life of fruits and vegetables when making a weekly meal plan, two shopping trips a week suffice to always have fresh products available with little loss in nutrients.

When using whole grain products, you have to adjust their preparation. Whole grain rice must be cooked in unsalted water otherwise it will not become soft. The same is the case with whole grain rice pudding. When cooking the rice in plain milk, it will not soften due to the mineral content of the milk. When I prepare rice pudding for desert, I first cook it in water; later I add some low-fat milk and finally a small amount of almond oil for aroma, which also adds the much desired ›good‹ fatty acids.«

Recipes for Transition, Fasting, and Building-up

The building-up phase is as important as fasting itself. This phase determines if the shift toward a healthy and calorie-conscious nutrition will be successful. To support your efforts, Hubert Hohler provides you with delicious recipes, not only for the building-up phase but also for the transition days, and even for the actual fast. The quantities given serve one person.

Transition Days—Detox Days

» Transition days serve to tune the body for the fast. Only one sort of food is eaten (e.g., rice, fruit, or potatoes/vegetables) and table salt is omitted. During these days, you take in fewer calories than usual and eliminate excess salt and water. The weight reduction begins and the circulatory system is relieved. The body is gently prepared for the fast. Step by step, the metabolism switches to fat burning and the »detoxification« during the first days of the fast brings less or no complications.

One pre-cleansing day should begin every fast. In a »deficient« constitution, where the person is exhausted, fatigued, pale, and tends to have low body weight, we recommend that the pre-cleansing phase is extended to 2 to 3 days.

Detox Days in Everyday Life

A »transition day« in everyday life is called a »detox day.« Pausing food intake once in a while is very popular nowadays and for a good reason. We should take every opportunity to eat less, whether it is through »dinner-canceling,« or periods of time (days or longer) with reduced caloric intake. The rejuvenating and anti-aging effect is caused by the immediate change in the hormonal balance. This is documented in numerous studies.

You will maintain your ideal weight more easily if you introduce 1 detox day per week. If you have eaten excessively, in a restaurant or at a party, you can counteract the results with a detox day. The excess calories are used immediately and possible water retention is resolved.

The same is true after an indigestive meal, when the tongue is coated, or with stomach ache or flatulence. In these cases, for example, a rice day could alleviate the discomfort. Colonic irrigation may be of additional help to restore healthy intestinal flora. When trying to balance a sumptuous meal, a fruit day usually works best. In cases of a sensitive stomach, sour fruits, such as pineapples and citrus fruits, should be avoided and stewed or soft fruit, like grapes, pears, or bananas, are preferable. In cases of diarrhea a banana day can work miracles. Diabetics should choose potato, oat, or protein days.

Fruit Day (ca. 600 kcal)

Eat 1.5 kg fresh fruit in three to four meals during the course of the day. You may use apples, pears, grapes, berries, and other ordinary seasonal fruits, but also exotic fruits, such as kiwis, mangos, papaya, and so on. This suggestion is only for people who tolerate fruits well.

People with sensitive gastro-intestinal tracts should choose a rice or oat day, and should at all cost avoid pineapple or sour fruits. A banana day (six to seven medium-sized bananas during the course of the day) can be very helpful if a tendency to diarrhea is present.

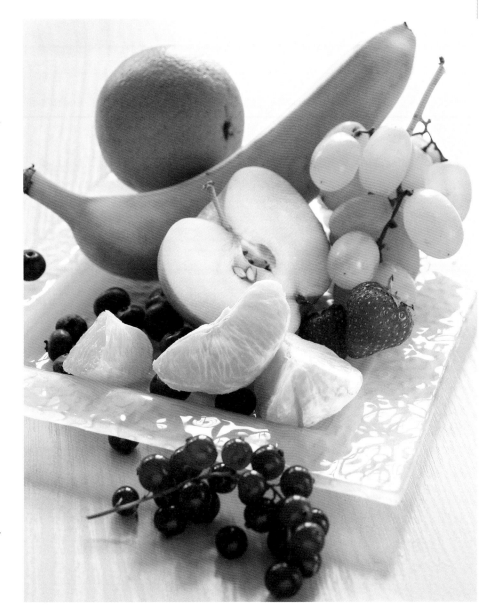

Rice Day (ca. 750 kcal)

To everyone unable to tolerate fruit generally or in large quantities, a rice day may be an alternative. Eat brown rice three times a day, which you can prepare sweet or savory.

Basic Rice Recipe

Ingredients: 150 mL water, 50 g brown rice, 1 bay leaf

- Rinse the rice under running water, place it in a pan with water and the bay leaf, bring to a boil then simmer covered for 30 minutes.

Savory Variation 1

Ingredients: ½ small onion, chopped, 1 small zucchini (courgette) (100 g), 2 tomatoes, pepper, garlic, 1 tbsp basil, chopped

- Sauté onions in a non-stick pan on medium heat until glazed. Cube zucchini, ca. 1 cm, add to the onions and sauté another 4 minutes. Cut each tomato into eight pieces, add to the pan and continue sautéing for an additional 4 minutes. Season with pepper and minced garlic to taste. Add basil before serving.

Savory Variation 2

Ingredients: 1 small onion, cubed, 500 g ripe tomatoes, sage, thyme (twig), pepper, 1 tbsp basil, chopped

- Sauté diced onions, without fat, on medium heat; cube tomatoes, ca. 1 cm, add to the pan with sage and thyme. Simmer for ca. 30 minutes; add pepper to taste and sprinkle with basil.

Sweet Variation

Ingredients: 1 medium-size apple (200 g), 1 pinch of cinnamon

- Quarter the apple and remove the core. Cut into thin slices. Sauté the apple slices in a non-stick pan on medium heat until soft. Add a little water if they lack moisture. Sprinkle with cinnamon. Add to 50 g of cooked rice.

Plating

Press the rice into a ring-shaped mold and turn it out on the plate, place the vegetable or fruit in the center.

Oat Day (ca. 550 kcal)

An oat day is recommendable in cases of sensitive stomach or diabetes mellitus. Three times a day you eat oat porridge with fruit. Briefly simmer 35 g of ground whole-grain oats in some water until they have a pastelike consistency. Add ca. 100 g of fruit (apple, berries, nectarine, apricot, etc.) or serve on the side.

Potato Day (ca. 800 kcal)

Divide 600 to 700 g of potatoes between three meals. The potatoes should be baked or boiled in the skin and served with fresh herbs, for example, thyme or caraway seeds. You may add 100 to 150 g of steamed vegetables per meal.

▶ Potato day/dinner: baked potato with lightly sautéed vegetables.

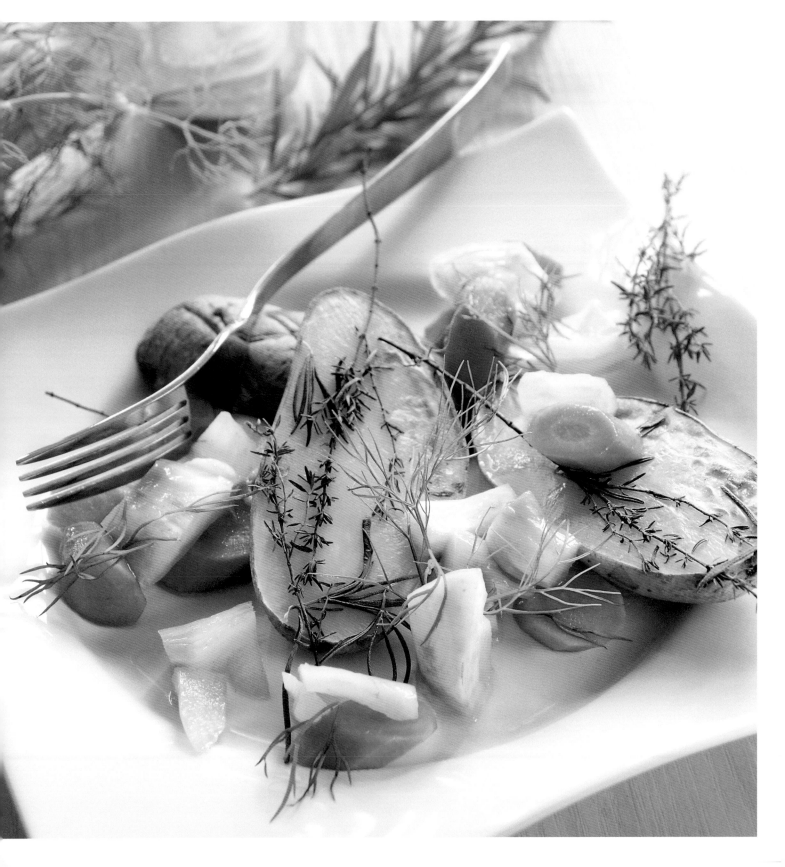

Breakfast

Ingredients: 1 medium-size potato (150 g), 1 small zucchini (courgette) (80 g), 1 tomato (80 g), rosemary twig, thyme twig, 1 tsp chopped basil

- Steam potato with the skin.
- Cut zucchini in half lengthwise and then cut into 1-cm slices. Place into a non-stick pan with the thyme and rosemary. Cook on medium heat for ca. 4 minutes and then add the sliced tomato. Cook for another 4 minutes. Finally, add the chopped basil and serve with the potato.

Lunch

Ingredients: 1 medium-size potato (150 g), 50 mL low-fat milk or soy milk, 1 pinch of nutmeg, freshly ground, 1 small onion, 300 g fresh spinach, rinsed and cleaned, nutmeg, pepper

- Steam potato with the skin, peel, mash with the potato ricer, and mix with warm milk and nutmeg. (Do not add salt or fat to the mashed potato.)
- Finely dice onion and sauté in a non-stick pan without oil. Add spinach and some water; close the lid and continue sautéing on medium heat for ca. 3 minutes.
- Add pepper and nutmeg to taste and serve the spinach with the mashed potato.

Dinner

Ingredients: 2 medium-size potatoes (300 g), 1 tsp herbs (rosemary, thyme), 1 fennel bulb, 1 carrot, 1 tsp chopped dill, pepper

- Wash and halve potatoes. Sprinkle rosemary and thyme on a baking sheet, place potatoes on top, and make cross-wise incisions in the skin. Bake for ca. 25 minutes at 170°C.
- Cut vegetables into 1-cm slices and sauté in a non-stick pan on medium heat for ca. 10 minutes. Add some water if necessary and finally season with dill and pepper.

Protein Day

Breakfast

Ingredients: 200 g cottage cheese, unsalted, 1 tsp rucola (rocket), pepper, ½ cucumber, 1 tomato

- Blend cottage cheese, rucola, and pepper until smooth. Cut cucumber and tomato into bite-size pieces and serve with cottage cheese mix.

Lunch

Ingredients: 80 g low-fat curd, 1 egg-white, 1 tsp basil, 1 pinch of curry powder, 1 pinch of paprika powder

- Blend all ingredients and pour into soufflé mold or cup. Cook for 15 minutes with steam or bain-marie: place the soufflé mold(s) in an ovenproof pan filled with water and bake at 160°C. Or, place the mold(s) in a pot or pan filled with water, cover and cook the soufflés on top of the stove on medium heat.

Ingredients: 1 small onion, 300 g fresh spinach, rinsed and cleaned, nutmeg, pepper

- Finely dice onion, sauté lightly in a non-stick pan, add spinach and some water, cover and sauté on medium heat for ca. 3 minutes.

- Add nutmeg and pepper to taste and serve with the soufflé.

Dinner

Ingredients: 200 g low-fat curd, 1 tsp chives, chopped, 1 tsp cilantro (coriander) powder, 2 tomatoes, 1 carrot

- Blend low-fat curd, chives, and cilantro until smooth, add some mineral water, if necessary. If you use carbonated water, the blend becomes foamier.
- Cut vegetables into bite-size pieces and serve with the curd.

Tip

You can also use fish for protein. Sauté the fish without adding fat or salt.

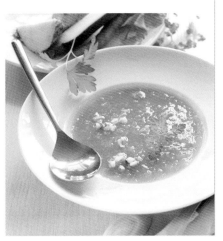

◄ Carrot and potato soup.

Vegetable Broth for the Fast

Ingredients: 300 mL water, 250 g vegetables (e.g., carrot, leek, onion, tomato, potato), 1 pinch of salt, 1 tbsp fresh herbs

- Peel and chop vegetables and add to the water; bring to a boil. Reduce heat and simmer on lowest heat for 15 to 30 minutes. Strain ca. 80% of the vegetables, purée the rest. Add a pinch of salt and serve the consommé with fresh herbs.

Tip

You can use any vegetable and combination of vegetables. This vegetable consommé is well suited for portioning and freezing.

Carrot and Potato Soup for the Evening when Breaking the Fast

Brunoise

Ingredients: 10 g carrots, 10 g zucchini (courgette)

- Finely dice (ca. 2-mm cubes), sauté al dente, and set aside.

Soup

Ingredients: 1 medium-size potato (80 g), 40 g carrots, 40 g leek, 40 g celery root, 40 g zucchini (courgette), 1 tsp butter (5 g), 300 mL water, 2–3 stalks of fresh herbs, such as parsley, chervil, marjoram, or lovage, 1 pinch of nutmeg, salt

- Wash and peel vegetables and cut into chunks. Place in a pot, add butter, and sauté lightly for some minutes on low heat. Stir with a wooden spatula to ensure that the vegetables are covered evenly with the fat. Add water and salt. Cover and let simmer for ca. 30 minutes. Purée vegetables with a hand-mixer and blend with some water if necessary. Add salt and nutmeg to taste.
- Add the brunoise, sprinkle with fresh herbs, such as parsley, chervil, marjoram, or lovage, and serve hot.

First Building-up Day

Breakfast:
Quinoa Apple Puree

Ingredients: 250 mL water, 30 g quinoa, shredded, 1 medium-size apple (200 g), 1 pinch of cinnamon, 1 tsp apple concentrate, 1 pinch of salt

- Bring the water to a boil, add the quinoa and return to a boil. Grate the apple finely, add to the quinoa and let it simmer for 5 minutes. Add the apple concentrate and spices to taste.

KNOWLEDGE

What is Quinoa?

Quinoa was the miraculous grain of the Incas and Mayas. It is gluten-free, very rich in minerals, not over-processed, and contains very little allergenic potential. This makes it an ideal food to re-start the gastrointestinal tract after a fast.

Lunch: Creamy Potato Puree with Fresh Spinach

Potato Puree

Ingredients: 1 medium-size potato, »mealy« (100 g), 25 mL whole milk, 1 tsp butter (5 g), salt, nutmeg

- Steam the potato in its skin and then peel it. Press the potato through the potato ricer. Melt the butter in the milk and bring to a boil. Whisk milk and potato and add spices. Press the blend through a pastry tube onto the plate, forming a V or B and place the spinach in the center.

Fresh Spinach

Ingredients: 150 g fresh spinach, ½ tsp olive oil (2 g), 1 clove of garlic, ½ small onion, chopped, vegetable broth, salt, nutmeg

- Remove spinach stalks and rinse thoroughly. Crush garlic clove and lightly sauté with the onion and olive oil in a pot. Add spinach and vegetable broth. Leave in the hot pot until spinach »wilts.« Season with salt and some nutmeg.
- You may also blanch the spinach in a steamer and then sauté it in olive oil and season.

Belgian Endive Salad in Cocktail Dressing

Rosy Yoghurt Dressing

Ingredients for 4 servings: 40 g yoghurt, 40 g sour cream, 40 g butter milk, ½ tsp freshly ground horseradish (1 g), 1 tbsp orange juice, freshly squeezed (5 g), 1 tbsp organic ketchup (15 g), salt

- Place all ingredients of the dressing into a bowl and blend well. If necessary add some seasoning.

Salad

Ingredients: 1 Belgian endive (50 g), 10 g radicchio, endive, green salad

- Set 4 endive leaves aside. Cut the rest of the endive in halves, remove the stalk, and cut all salad leaves into fine strips. Arrange salad on a plate, decorate with the 4 endive leaves, and dress with the cocktail sauce.

▶ Belgian endive salad with cocktail dressing.

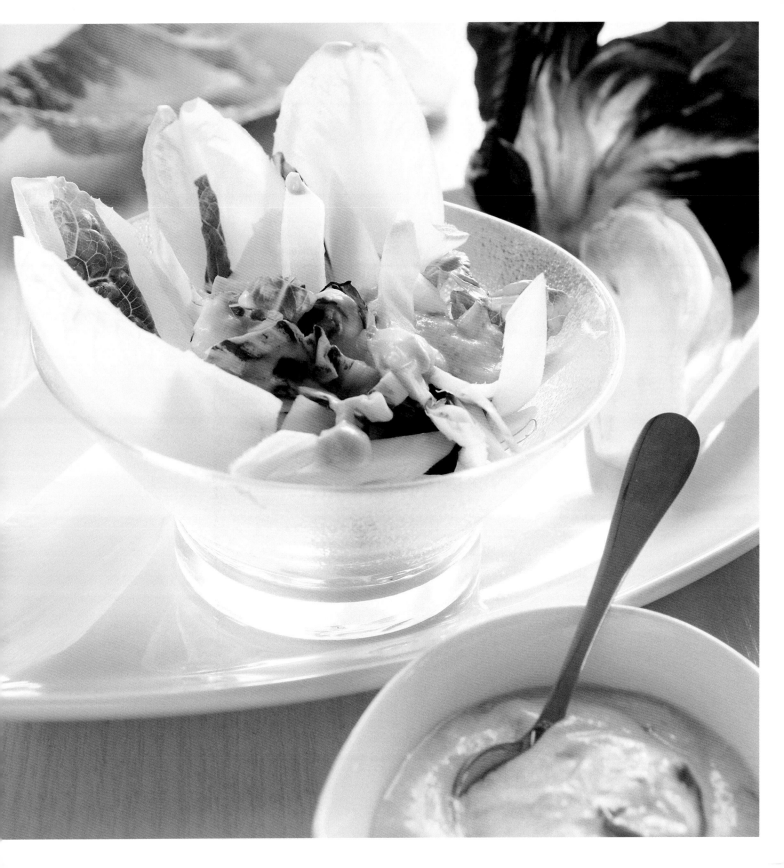

Dinner: Tender Fennel Hearts in Dressing

Ingredients: 3 tbsp freshly squeezed orange juice (30 g), 1 tsp almond oil (5 g), a dash of raspberry vinegar, 1 fennel bulb (100 g), finely grated, 20 g orange, fresh (for decoration), salt

- Blend the ingredients for the dressing, take out the fennel heart and cut into wafer-thin strips or grate directly into the dressing. The fennel should marinate in the dressing for 30 minutes to be well infused. Salt to taste and decorate with orange slices.

Vegetable Potpourri in a Golden Yellow Saffron Sauce

Ingredients: 15 g whole grain rice, 1 bay leaf, vegetable broth, 60 g pumpkin, olive oil, ginger, finely grated, 1 pinch of curry powder, 60 g zucchini (courgette), 30 g sugar snaps, rosemary, garlic, salt, pepper, 30 g sauce, basic recipe (see recipe p. 145), ½ tsp almond oil (2 g), 1 pinch of saffron

Rice

- Cook the rice with the bay leaf covered in 2½ times the amount of unsalted vegetable broth for ca. 30 minutes until tender. Before serving, add olive oil and sea salt to taste.

Vegetables

- Cube the pumpkin, lightly sauté in some olive oil and add the finely grated ginger. Season with curry powder, salt, and pepper; add some broth and sauté on low heat until tender.
- Slice the zucchini, cut the ends of the sugar snaps, pull off the strings, if necessary, and steam al dente.
- Toss zucchini slices in a pan with rosemary, salt, pepper, a small amount of garlic, and olive oil. Also sauté sugar snaps lightly in olive oil; season to taste.

Sauce

- Follow the basic recipe for the sauce. Add saffron and blend in the almond oil. Shortly before serving, mix again with the hand-held blender.

Plating

Pour the sauce on a plate, press the rice in a mold and carefully turn it out on the plate. Arrange vegetables in a color-coordinated pattern on the plate.

▶ Vegetable potpourri in a golden-yellow saffron sauce.

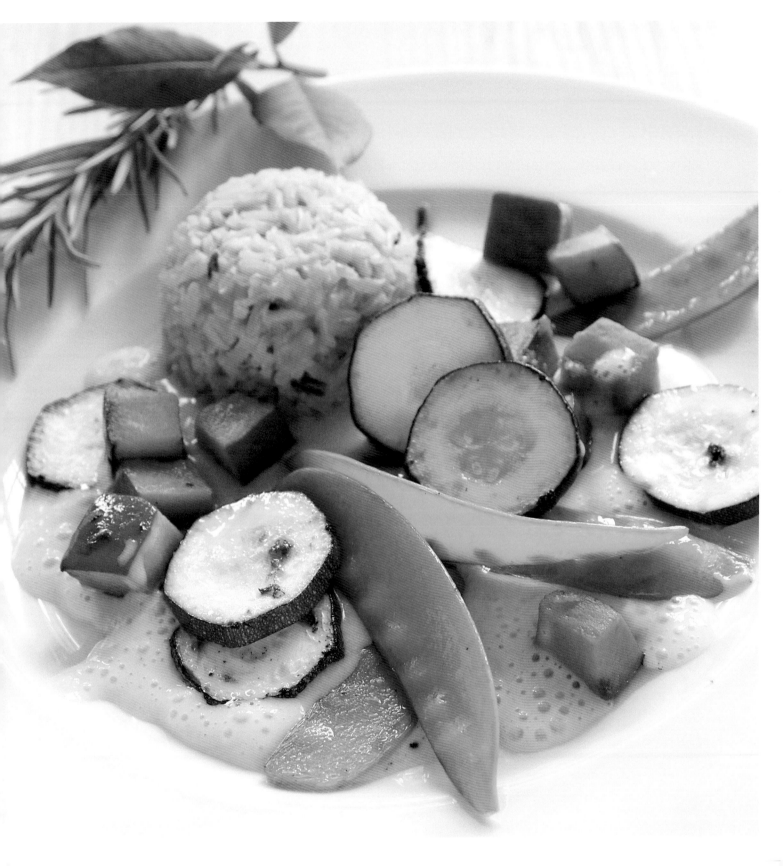

Second Building-up Day

Breakfast: Budwig Cream by Dr. Kousmine

Ingredients: 40 g low-fat curd, 1 tsp flax seed oil (4 g), ½ to 1 banana (50 g), orange or lemon juice as needed, 1 tbsp grains (e.g., oats, 10 g), finely ground, 1 apple, 1 tbsp oilseeds (e.g., flax seeds, 10 g), soaked or crushed, 30 g fruit of the season

- Blend curd and flax seed oil, purée banana and mix in, add juice and ground grains.
- Cut the apple in half, and grate it after removing the core. Add apple and oilseeds to the blend.
- Decorate with fruits of the season.

KNOWLEDGE

Budwig Cream

The Budwig cream is a classic. It was composed by Dr. Catherine Kousmine in honor of Dr. Johanna Budwig, who understood the paramount importance of cold-pressed linseed oil and omega-3 fatty acids and the danger of hydrogenated fats. It features a handy meal that contains the majority of nutrients we need every day. Ingredients, such as low-fat curd, flax seed oil, fresh fruit, nuts, and some grain, provide many vital substances and yet contain few calories.

Lunch: Green Salad with Sprouts in Avocado Cream Sauce

Ingredients: 60 g green salad leaves (seasonal), 20 g sprouts

- Rinse salad leaves and chop into smaller pieces. Rinse and drain sprouts. Arrange salad on a plate and sprinkle sprouts over the salad or mix them in.

Avocado Cream Sauce

Ingredients (serves 4): 20 mL apple vinegar, 100 mL water, 1 tsp mustard, 50 mL cold-pressed walnut oil, ¼ avocado (50 g), 1 garlic clove, crushed, salt, pepper, 1 tbsp freshly chopped herbs

- Purée all ingredients, except the herbs, in a blender until creamy. Add the finely chopped herbs last. Arrange green salad leaves on a plate, sprinkle sprouts over the salad and dress with the avocado sauce.

Quinoa Soufflé, Tomato with Eggplant Caviar

Ingredients: 20 g quinoa, cooked (net weight 9 g), water, 80 g low-fat curd, ½ whisked egg, 1 tsp grated parmesan (3 g), herb salt, nutmeg, 1 tsp parsley, ½ tsp olive oil to grease the mold (1 g)

Quinoa Soufflé

- Cook quinoa in double the amount of water. Set aside to cool.
- Blend cooled grain with low-fat curd, egg, and grated cheese. Fold in parsley. Add herb salt and nutmeg to taste.
- Pour the batter into an oiled mold and let it cook or thicken for 20 minutes in a bain-marie or in the oven (medium heat).

▶ Green salad with sprouts in avocado cream sauce.

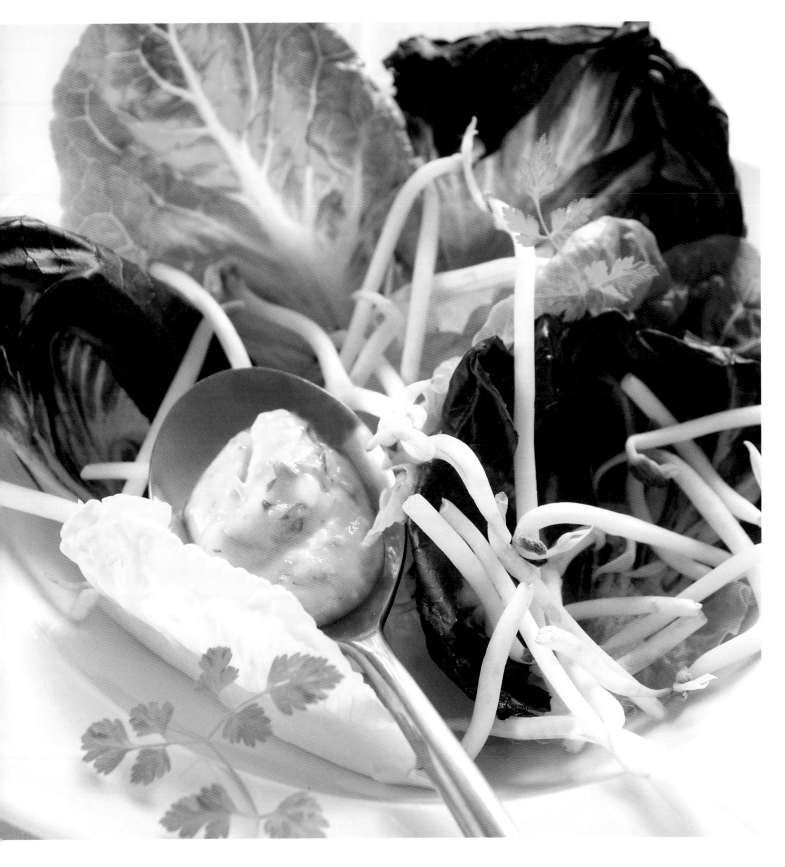

Tomato with Eggplant Caviar

Ingredients: 1 eggplant (aubergine), ½ small onion, finely diced, ½ tsp olive oil, chives, rosemary, salt, pepper, 1 to 2 tomatoes (100 g), salt, pepper, 3 g grated parmesan

- Cut eggplant in half. Cook in the oven at 200°C, scrape out with a spoon and chop finely. Lightly sauté the onion and garlic in olive oil, add the finely chopped eggplant caviar, blend in herbs and season.
- Cut tomatoes in half, season with salt and pepper, place eggplant caviar on top and bake for 15 minutes at 170°C. Sprinkle with the parsley.

Zucchini Sauce

Ingredients: ½ zucchini (courgette) (35 g), ½ onion (20 g), 1 rosemary twig, salt and pepper

- Dice zucchini and onion and brown with the rosemary in a pan; add 50 mL water and sauté until tender.
- Season with salt and pepper and purée.

Dinner: Potatoes in the Skin with Budwig Cream and Beetroot Crescents

Ingredients: 2 potatoes in the skin (180 g) steamed

Budwig Cream

Ingredients: 100 g low-fat curd, 1 tsp flax seed oil (5 g), 1 tsp sunflower seeds (5 g), 1 tsp freshly chopped herbs (e.g., dill, parsley to taste), salt

- Whisk curd until smooth, add the flax seed oil and whisk until oil has completely emulsified. Now add sunflower seeds and herbs. Salt to taste. Fold in everything once more.

Beetroot Crescents

Ingredients: 1 small beetroot (40 g), 150 mL beetroot juice, 1 tsp rice flour (5 g)

- Cut the beetroot into 8 equal wedges, place in beetroot juice and cook until tender. To thicken the juice for serving, pour the rice flour into the boiling liquid, continuously stirring, and let it cook for 2 more minutes.
- Plate the beetroot and coat with the sauce, add the potato in the skin and serve with the Budwig cream.

Zucchini Salad in Creamy Dill Sauce

Ingredients: 1 medium-size zucchini (courgette), 1 tsp olive oil, cold-pressed (3 g), 1 tsp vinegar (3 g) or lemon juice, 1 tsp chopped parsley, 1 pinch of salt

- Rinse the zucchini and cut it into wafer-thin slices without peeling it. Place it into the marinade made of olive oil, vinegar or lemon juice, chopped parsley and salt.

Dill Sauce

Ingredients: 1 tbsp yoghurt (1.5% fat) (10 g), 1 tbsp buttermilk (5 g), 1 tsp mustard (2 g), 1 tsp fresh dill (2 g), salt, pepper

- Blend all ingredients for the dill sauce in a bowl until creamy, salt and pepper to taste.
- Arrange zucchini on a plate and dress with seasonal salads and the dill sauce.

▶ Potatoes in the skin with Budwig cream and beetroot crescents.

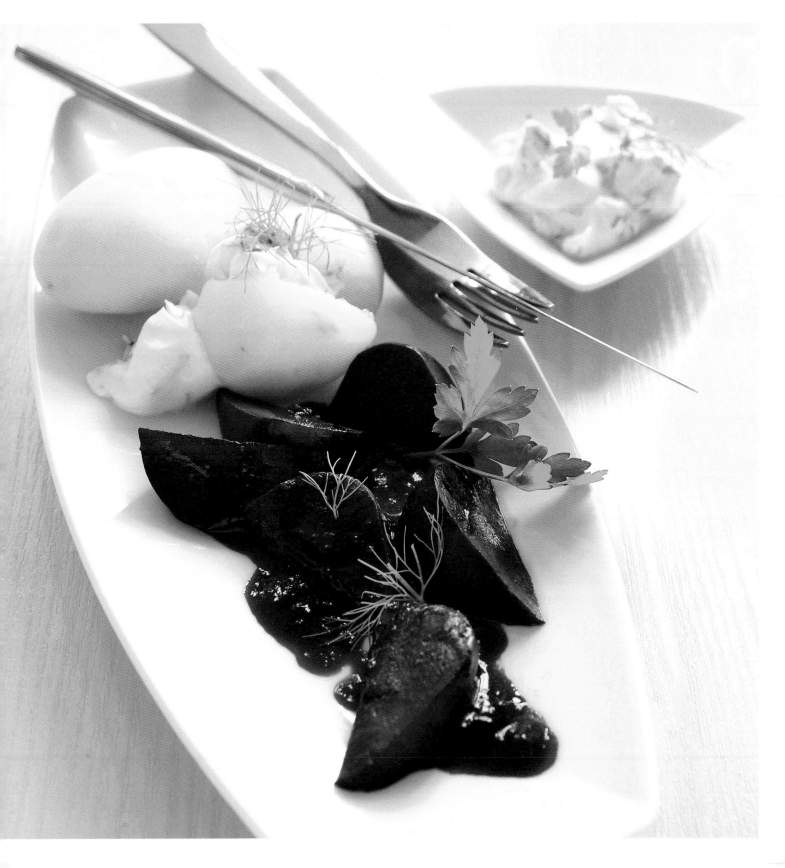

Third Building-up Day

Breakfast: Budwig Cream

The recipe for the Budwig cream has been introduced on page 120. You may vary the added fruits or grains according to your personal preferences.

Lunch: Sauerkraut Salad

Ingredients: 80 g sauerkraut, 1 tsp olive oil (5 g), 1 tsp apple juice, chopped herbs (chives, marjoram, parsley), 50 g leaf salad, 2 tbsp vinaigrette (see basic recipe p. 145)

- Spread out the sauerkraut a little, if necessary cut it into smaller pieces and marinate it in the olive oil, apple juice, and herbs.
- Arrange on a plate with the leaf salad and dress with the vinaigrette.

Belgian Endive with Bulgur

Ingredients: 500 mL water, 1 bay leaf, 1 Belgian endive, 1 tsp salt, pepper, whole grain flour, olive oil, 50 g carrots, zucchini (courgette), 40 g diced tomatoes, 20 g bulgur, dry (or 40 g cooked), chervil, chives, salt, pepper, 35 g white basic sauce, 1 tsp walnut oil (5 g), ½ tsp parsley, chopped, 1 tbsp parmesan (3 g)

- Bring water with bay leaf to a boil. Place Belgian endive into the boiling water and let it simmer for 30 minutes.
- Remove Belgian endive from water and drain, lightly press flat and season with salt and pepper. Dredge in the whole grain flour. On medium heat, brown in a pan with some olive oil until golden.
- Cook bulgur with double the amount of water.
- Finely dice carrots and zucchini and lightly sauté in olive oil. Add tomato cubes and bulgur. Season with herbs and spices.
- Bring the basic sauce to a boil, add walnut oil and blend. Add parsley for well-rounded taste.

Plating

Pour sauce on a plate and arrange Belgian endive on top. Press bulgur mix into a ladle and turn out on to the plate, sprinkle with parmesan before serving.

Dinner: Celery in Apple–Orange Jus

Ingredients: 60 g celery, 20 g apple, 20 g orange, 1 tsp walnut oil (5 g), 1 tsp orange juice (5 g), salt, pepper, 50 g leaf salad, 2 tbsp vinaigrette (see basic recipe p. 145)

- Peel fibers off the celery stalk, or peel stalk with a potato peeler, cut in thin slices and marinate in walnut oil, orange juice, finely chopped apple and orange, salt and pepper.
- Arrange celery with leaf salad on a plate and dress with the vinaigrette.

Aromatic Vegetable Millet Soufflé

Ingredients: 2 medium-size carrots (200 g), 50 g leek, 1 egg, cilantro (coriander) stalk, thyme twig, salt, pepper, 20 g millet (cooked), 60 g carrots, 60 g seasonal vegetables, 35 g basic sauce (see basic recipe p. 145), 1 tsp almond oil (5 g), 1 tsp dill (3 g)

- Steam cook carrots and leek, set aside to cool. Purée with the egg and season with salt and pepper. Add cooked millet and fill soufflé molds.
- Cook for 15 minutes in bain-marie or steam.
- Prepare the sauce according to the basic recipe and blend with almond oil. Just before serving, mix again with the hand-mixer and add dill.

▶ Preparing Belgian endive with bulgur is a little more time-consuming, as the Belgian endive should cook for 30 minutes.

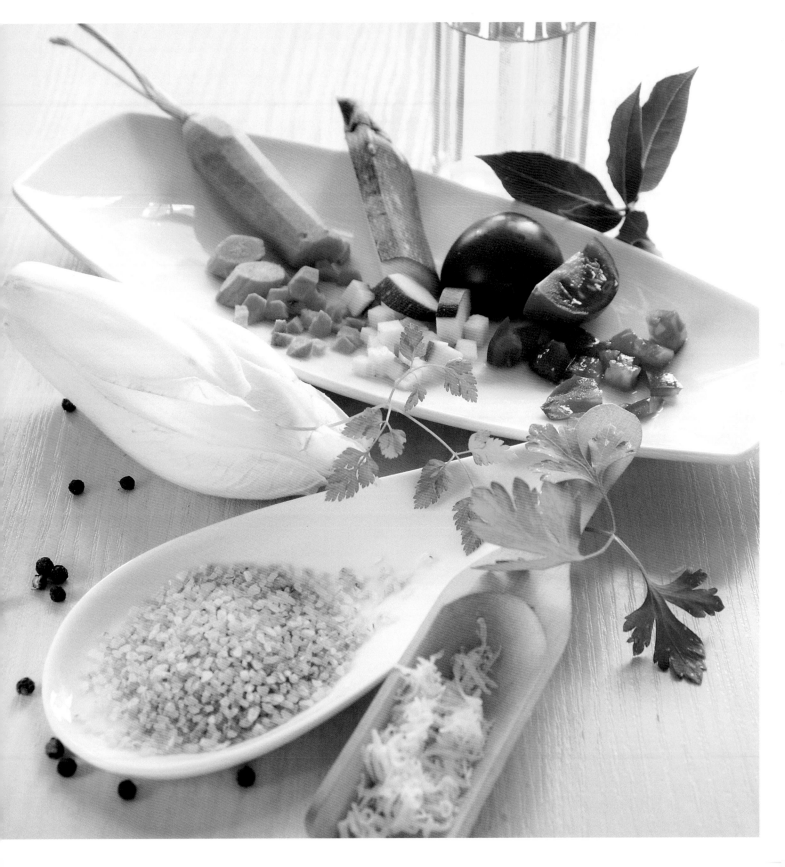

Eating Healthily after the Fast

Make your nutrition after the fast the new beginning of a healthy whole food diet. In the conversation with Hubert Hohler (pp 106–109) we have already touched on some central issues, such as sensitization of taste, the proper use of oils, and the careful preparation of vegetables. On the following pages I will explain the fundamentals of a whole food diet, which keeps you in good health and is ideal to maintain weight.

Diet is the art of taking in the proper amount of nutrients without overtaxing the digestive tract. The most important recommendations include:

- Only eat when you are truly hungry. Stop eating as soon as you are full.
- You notice in time that the slower you eat, the sooner you are full. You may miss the point of fullness more easily when you eat too quickly.
- Only eat foods that you can digest and metabolize without difficulties.
- Learn not to compensate emotional deficiency with eating. Develop adequate coping strategies.

Natural foods, including fruit, vegetables, nuts, legumes, and whole grains are high in vitamins, minerals, secondary plant compounds, essential fatty acids, and valuable proteins. This makes them highly recommended. Nevertheless, especially as raw foods, they are not digestible equally by everyone and may cause fermentation and putrefaction processes in some people. Pay attention to body signals to find your individual limits of tolerance. Preferably buy certified organic products.

Choosing Proper Fats

» Vegetable fats from nuts and oil seeds, as well as cold-pressed oils, are highly valuable because they are high in mono- and polyunsaturated fatty acids. These fatty acids are essential, that is, vital, as the body cannot generate them and depends on the external supply. They belong to the omega-3 and omega-6 families.

KNOWLEDGE

What about Butter?

Butter (milk fat) is a natural product that is high in cholesterol and saturated fatty acids. This is why excessive milk fat consumption is responsible for several modern diseases (e.g., cardiovascular diseases).

There is nothing wrong with moderate consumption of milk fat (20 to 30 g per day) if the entire fat consumption is limited to an average of 60 to 80 g per day. Keep in mind that butter, milk, cream, and cheese contain milk fat and by the end of the day it can add up to a considerable amount. Low-fat dairy products (low-fat curd, buttermilk, 1.5% fat yoghurt) help to reduce fat consumption.

Milk fat content in various products (per 100 g):
- 100 g butter contains   ca. 80 to 90 g milk fat
- 100 g cheese contains   ca. 10 to 40 g milk fat (depending on the type)
- 100 g cream contains   ca. 30 g milk fat
- 100 g whole milk contains ca. 3.5 g milk fat

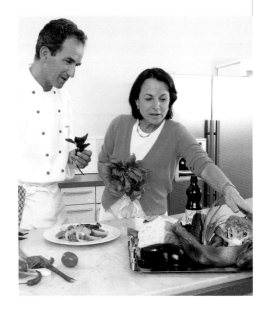

▲ »Non-heated foods,« such as salads, raw foods, and fresh fruits, are well suited to begin a meal, as they stimulate digestive processes. In addition, these foods are particularly recommended because they are low in calories but high in nutritional value and saturation effect. They are the true »light« products!

The daily requirement of polyunsaturated fatty acids is easily covered, for example, with 1 to 2 tablespoons of cold-pressed sunflower oil and 2 teaspoons cold-pressed flax-seed oil. In addition, olive oil and nuts, as well as some milk fat (butter, cream, or cheese) are recommended, provided that your weight allows it.

Fats that must be entirely avoided include margarine, hydrogenated fats, frying and deep-frying fats, as well as conventional (refined) oils.

Preferably Use Whole-Grain Products

» In contrast to white flour products, whole-grain flour is high in valuable substances that the organism requires: protein, polyunsaturated fatty acids, carbohydrates, vitamins (B-complex in particular), minerals, and last but not least dietary fibers (e.g., bran). If possible, the grain should be freshly ground or cracked.

Buying a grain mill is recommended.

The following grains are available almost everywhere: wheat, rice, rye, oat, barley, millet, corn, unripe spelt, spelt, buckwheat, quinoa, and amaranth. Make sure that the grain is also certified organically grown! It is recommended that you introduce at least one whole food meal per day, for example, Budwig cream by Dr. Kousmine (see recipe p. 120).

Eat Plenty of Fruits and Vegetables

» Fruits and vegetables supply us primarily with vitamins, minerals, and carbohydrates, as well as dietary fibers and bioactive substances. Only products in their natural state contain these bioactive plant products. Food processing, for example, heating, destroys these vital substances that protect the heart, ward off cancer, and are anti-inflammatory. Examples of bioactive plant products include carotenoids, polyphenols, terpenes, phytoestrogens, or dietary fibers.

Raw foods must always be chewed well! If flatulence or indigestion occurs, the amount of raw food should be reduced or replaced by cooked vegetables, soups, or stewed fruits, which are significantly easier to digest.

Additional Recommendations

» Refined products (e.g., white flour and products made from it, semolina, starch flour, white rice, refined sugar) are processed more than once. Every time that they are processed their nutritional and saturation value decreases, because vital substances and dietary fiber is removed. Aside from their quickly resorbed carbohydrates, refined products are considered »depleted« constituents of our nutrition and their consumption should be deliberately reduced.

Reduce Meat Consumption

In principle, meat and fish are high-value foods. However, conventional livestock breeding with its hormone administration, medication treatments, as well as environmental influences on feeding, reduce the quality of meat. Generally, this also applies to fish. In addition, meat is high in cholesterol, saturated fatty acids, and purines that turn into uric acid when broken down in the human organism. If you wish to eat meat, it is recommended that you limit the consumption to 100 to 150 g per day, preferably eaten at lunch time. Only eat high-quality meat from good sources.

Choose fish over meat more frequently. In particular, the fish oil in ocean fish (herring, mackerel, and salmon) is high in omega-3 fatty acids, which lower the triglycerides and at the same time increase the »good« HDL cholesterol, preventing arteriosclerosis and cardiac infarction.

Alternatives to meat dishes include grain dishes, mushrooms, legumes, such as peas, beans, soy beans, and lentils, nuts, and oilseeds; milk, dairy products, and eggs depending on their digestibility.

Limit Alcohol Intake

From the perspective of nutritional science, the harmfulness of alcohol, especially on the nervous system, is a matter of dosage. Alcohol may have a positive stimulating effect in small quantities. Good wine also contains bioactive plant products that protect the heart.

Negative effects of alcohol include the inhibition of fat burning and the accumulation of fat deposits in the abdominal area.

Furthermore, alcohol stresses the liver during detoxification and carries large amounts of calories:
- 1 glass of wine (125 mL) = ca. 90 kcal
- 1 glass of beer (330 mL) = ca. 145 kcal
- 1 glass of spirits, for example, cognac/40% vol. (40 mL) = ca. 110 kcal

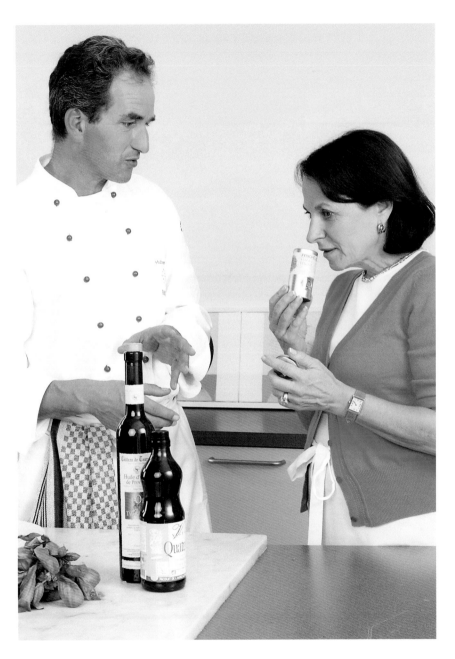

Little Salt

Table salt consumption should be limited to below 6 g per day, that is, the consumption of finished products, bread, and cheese must be curtailed. Make sure that you drink plenty of water, at least 1.5 L per day.

◀ A low-sodium diet should not be confused with a bland diet. You can experiment with spices and herbs, and discover the variety of ways one dish can taste, depending on the spicy notes you give it.

129

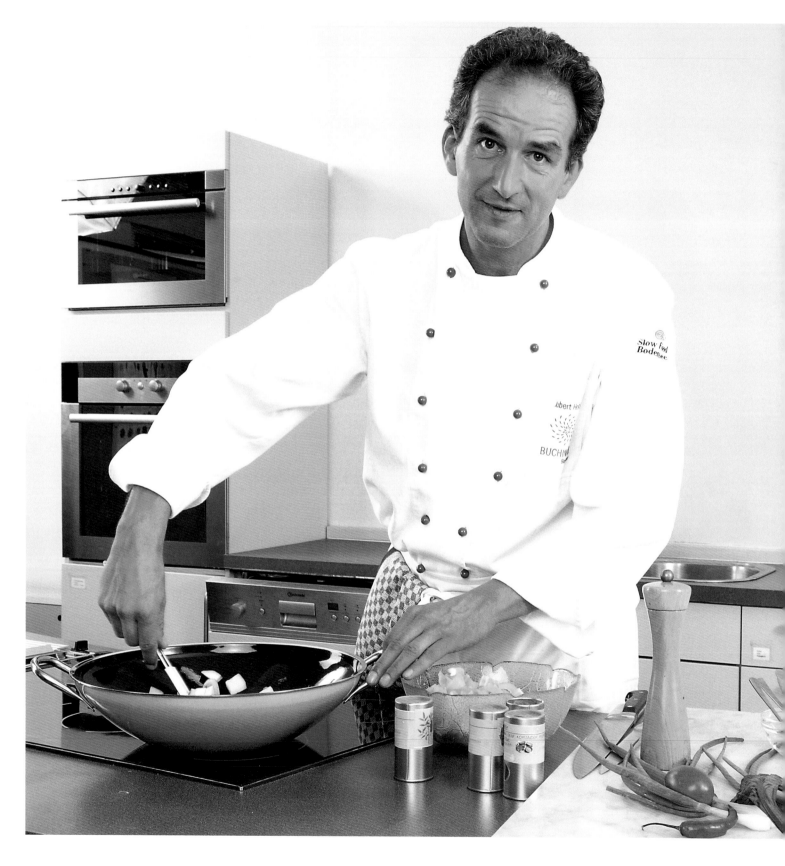

Recipes

In this section, you will find trusted recipes from the Buchinger clinic at Lake Constance that will help you to develop a diverse and balanced low-calorie diet rich in vital substances. We hope you enjoy experimenting and eating. Unless stated otherwise, the recipes serve two people.

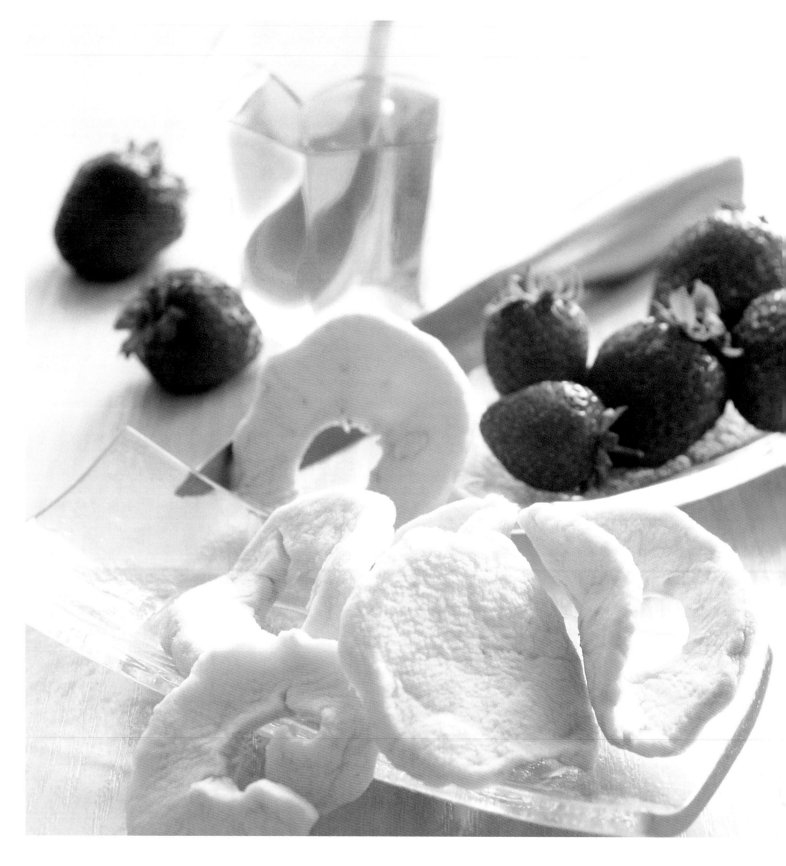

Healthy Ideas for Breakfast

Breakfast should supply you with the energy to start the day. Ideally, begin with muesli, for example, the Budwig cream (see recipe p. 120). The muesli tastes different every time if you vary the added fruit and grain types. Budwig cream can also be used as a spread, preferably on whole grain bread. I advise against ready-made breakfast cereals. They are processed and usually high in sugar or other sweeteners. Bread spreads are easy to make. Fruity or savory, simply try the recipes below. You will realize that a tasty bread spread does not require large amounts of fat or sugar.

Chocolate Spread

Ingredients: 250 mL milk, 3 tbsp cocoa powder, 1 pinch of vanilla, 1 pinch of salt, 30 g polenta (cornmeal), 50 g filberts (hazelnuts), finely ground, 1 tbsp almond oil (10 g), 60 g honey

- Bring milk with cocoa powder, vanilla, and salt to a boil.
- Stir polenta and ground filberts into boiling milk. Cook for 2 to 3 minutes until the mix turns into porridge. Stir honey and oil into the hot porridge, taste, and purée with a hand-held mixer. Pour into a glass, seal, and leave to cool.

◀ To make the spread, soak the sliced apple rings with the strawberries for a few hours.

Fruity Strawberry Apple Spread

Ingredients: 50 g dried apple rings, 200 g strawberries (fresh or frozen), honey as needed

- Cut apple rings into chunks and let them sit with the strawberries for a few hours, so the apple rings can soak up the juice. Purée and sweeten with honey if desired.

Tip

All ripe fruits may be used for this type of bread spread. The amount of dried fruits depends on the water content of the fruits.

This spread can be kept in the refrigerator for 1 week.

Red Lentil Spread

Ingredients: 1 onion (50 g), 1 carrot (125 g), 1 twig of marjoram, 1 tsp olive oil (5 g), 125 g red lentils, 1 tbsp tomato paste (15 g), 500 mL vegetable broth, 2 tbsp raspberry vinegar (20 g), 2 tbsp almond oil (20 g), salt, pepper

- Dice the onion, peel the carrot, and cut into small pieces; lightly sauté both in olive oil with the marjoram twig. Add red lentils, stir in tomato paste, and deglaze with the vegetable broth and raspberry vinegar. Continue to cook until all ingredients are soft. Place in a blender, add the almond oil, salt and pepper to taste, and purée.

Soups

Soups are a vital part of a fresh, healthy diet. They can be prepared simply and without taking a lot of time. When prepared properly, they supply us with a large amount of vegetables and enrich our diet.

Parsnip Coconut Soup

Ingredients: 1 parsnip (150 g), ½ leek (125 g), 1 small potato (50 g), ½ fennel bulb (70 g), 50 g desiccated coconut, 1 L vegetable broth, 50 mL milk, 1 tbsp almond oil (10 g), salt, cayenne pepper

- Cut vegetables into small pieces and lightly sauté together with the desiccated coconut, without using fat. Add vegetable broth and cook until soft. Put in a blender, add milk and almond oil, purée and season to taste.
- If desired, the soup may be strained to remove the desiccated coconut.

Vegetable Broth

Ingredients: 80 g onions, sliced, 400 g chopped root vegetables (carrots, celery, fennel), 1 clove of garlic, 1.5 L water, rosemary and thyme (1 twig each), 1 bay leaf, juniper berries, salt, pepper

- Lightly sauté vegetables and onion without using fat, add the garlic clove and heat briefly. Add the water.
- Add herbs and spices; continue to cook for ca. 1 hour, until vegetables are soft; strain and season.
- The consommé can be served with various additions (e.g., vegetables, meatballs, dumplings, or noodles) or used as a tasty liquid for cooking.

Pumpkin Lemongrass Soup

Ingredients: ½ small onion, 120 g pumpkin (e.g., Hokaido), lemongrass, ginger, ½ tsp curry powder, 400 mL vegetable broth or water, salt, pepper, 1 tbsp almond oil (10 g), raspberry vinegar

- Chop the onion and the pumpkin into walnut-sized pieces, lightly sauté together with the spices, without using fat; deglaze with the liquid. Continue to cook the vegetables until soft; purée in a blender until the soup is smooth and creamy. (Remove lemongrass before puréeing.)
- Salt and pepper to taste; add almond oil and raspberry vinegar, and mix again. If the soup is too thick, adjust consistency by adding vegetable broth or milk.

Tip

This soup may also be served cold.

▶ Pumpkin lemongrass soup

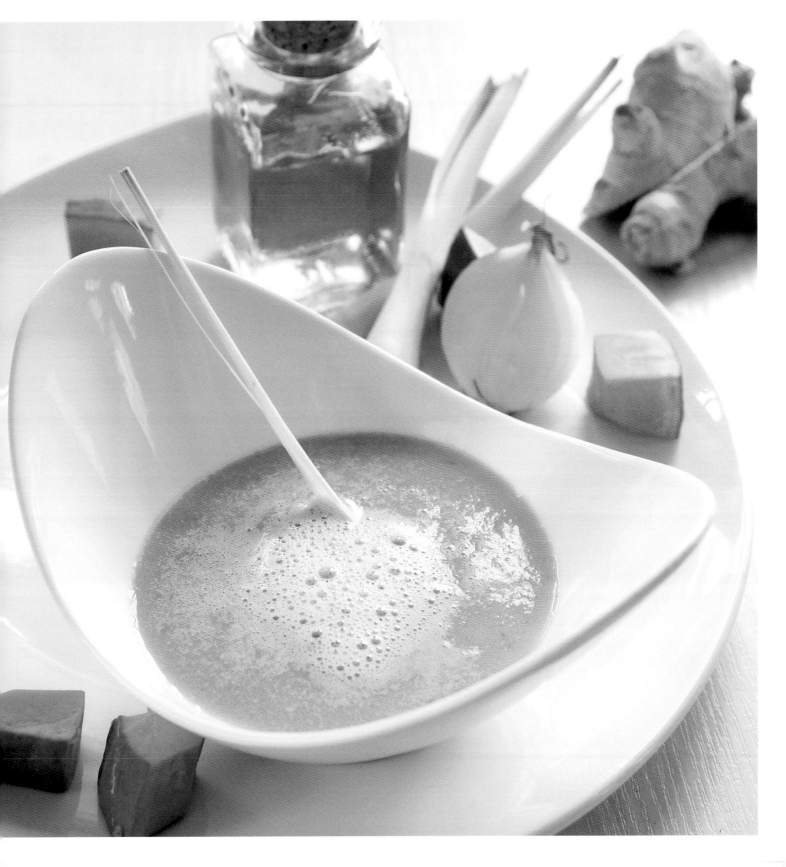

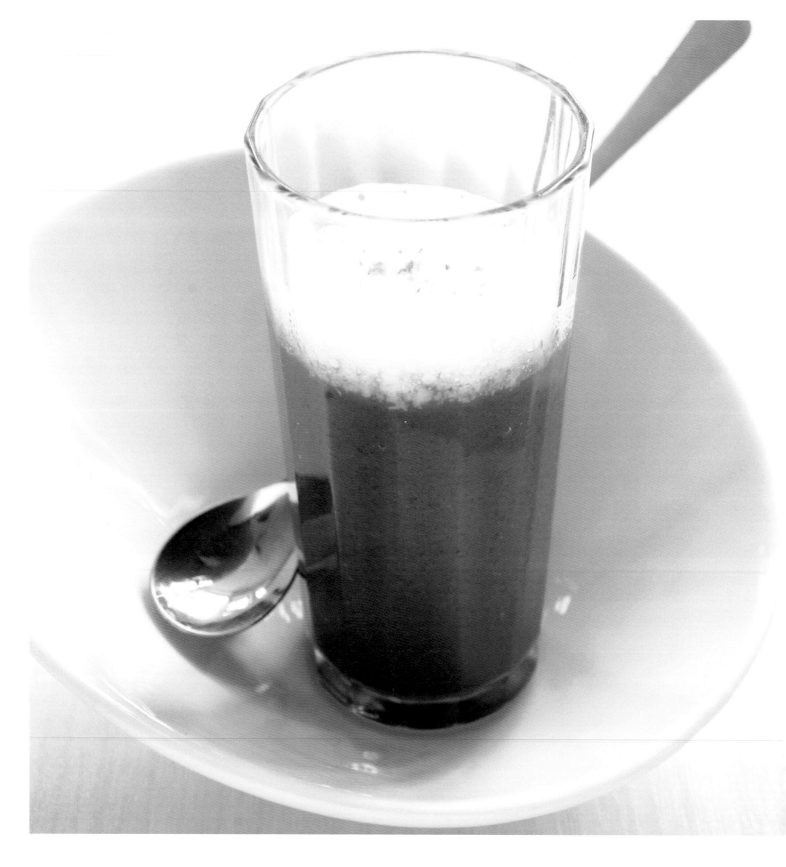

Beetroot Macchiato

Ingredients: 1 small beetroot (120 g), 1 small potato, peeled (50 g), 20 g leek, 1 tsp olive oil (5 g), 400 mL vegetable broth, 1 bay leaf, salt, pepper, 1 pinch of caraway, 1 tbsp walnut oil (10 g), 1 tbsp apple cider vinegar, 200 mL milk (1.5% fat), 1 tbsp freshly shredded horseradish, 1 pinch of Espelette pepper (French chili pepper, replaceable by some chili and paprika powder)

Vegetable Soup

- Chop beetroot and potato walnut size, slice leek finely, and lightly sauté the vegetables in olive oil.
- Add the vegetable broth and bay leaf, and simmer on low heat until soft.
- Remove the bay leaf when everything is soft and purée the soup in the blender. While puréeing, add the apple cider vinegar, the oil, and the spices (salt, pepper, and caraway) and taste.
- If the soup is too thick, adjust consistency by adding vegetable broth.

Froth

- Simmer milk, horseradish, and Espelette pepper for 5 minutes on low heat; strain and froth with a hand-held mixer or milk frother.
- If the milk is too hot it does not froth well.

Plating

Pour the soup into a glass and spoon the froth on top. Serve immediately.

Asparagus Soup

Ingredients: ½ small onion, 300 g asparagus, peeled, 2 small potatoes, peeled, 500 mL water, a small amount lemon juice, ¼ tsp salt, pepper, 1 tbsp walnut oil (10 g), 1 tsp tarragon or dill, chopped

- Slice the onion and lightly sauté in a pot on medium heat; chop potatoes and asparagus and add to the onion; sauté another 2 minutes, add the water and cook until soft.
- Remove asparagus tips and cut into small pieces. Purée remaining soup with oil and lemon juice in a blender. When finished, add the cut asparagus tips to the soup.
- Tarragon or dill complements the flavor of the soup.

◀ Beetroot macchiato

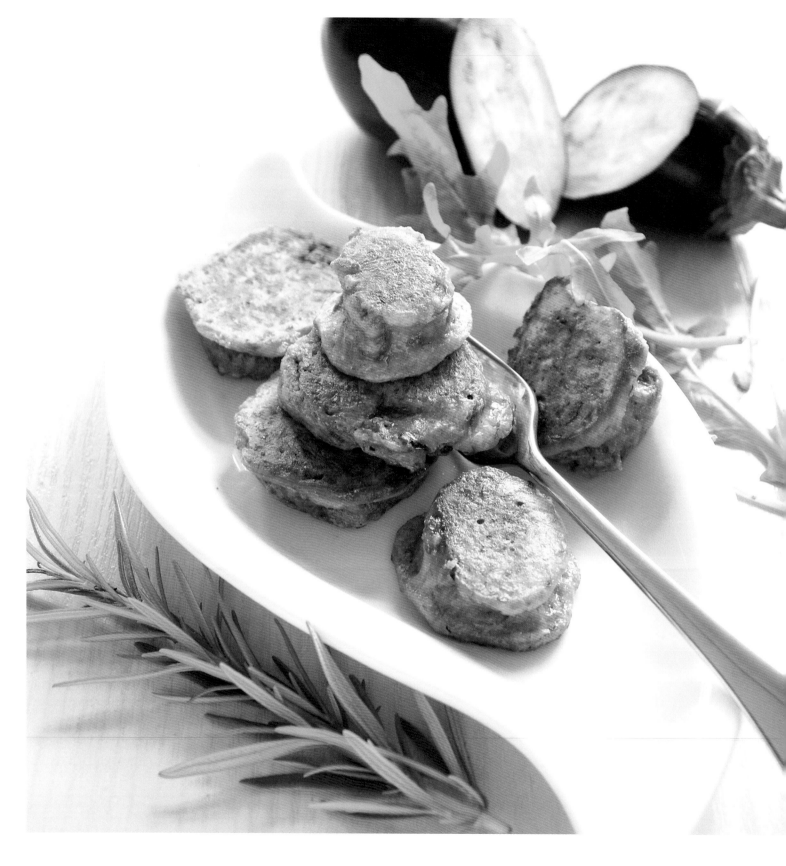

Savory Dishes

Many people would eat vegetarian meals more often if they had ideas for simple fast dishes. Everything new takes a little getting used to in the beginning, but with some practice you can handle the preparation of these dishes just like you do the familiar ones.

Eggplant Piccata

Ingredients: 22 g eggplant (aubergine), soy sauce, pepper, rosemary, 1 egg, 30 g whole grain flour, 40 mL milk, 1 tbsp rucola (rocket), chopped, 30 g parmesan, grated, salt, pepper, paprika powder, some whole grain flour for breading

- Prick the eggplants all the way around with a small knife (to prevent them from bursting when stewing in the oven) and place them on a baking-sheet or heat-resistant pan. Bake in the oven at 160°C until eggplants are soft (approximately 15 minutes).
- Peel off the skin (if the eggplants are soft the skin comes off easily), cut the eggplant in slices of ca. 1 cm, and season with soy sauce, pepper, and rosemary.
- Break the egg and whisk it, beat in the flour while stirring with a whisk. Fold in milk, parmesan, rucola, and spices.
- Bread the seasoned eggplant slices first with flour; dip them into the egg mix and fry them.

Tip

This type of piccata can also be made with kohlrabi or zucchini; the latter do not have to be pre-cooked. The cooked eggplants may also be breaded.

Side Dishes

Rice, spaghetti, or polenta (cornmeal) go well with this dish, as well as tomato sauce or tomato coulis (see recipe p. 147).

◀ Eggplant piccata

Cauliflower Curry

Ingredients: ½ tsp curry powder, 1 spring onion, ½ medium-size cauliflower (400 g), 100 mL water, 1 tbsp tamari (Japanese soy sauce) (10 g), 1 tsp roasted sesame oil (5 g), lemon juice, 1 tbsp cilantro (coriander) powder

- Heat curry powder in a frying pan, add chopped spring onion and cauliflower, add water, cover, and cook on medium heat for 15 minutes.
- Season with tamari, sesame oil, lemon juice, and cilantro powder.

HERE'S HOW IT'S DONE!

How to Brown the Piccata

Place up to 1 tablespoon of vegetable oil, suitable for high-temperature cooking, and ½ teaspoon of water in a non-stick frying pan. As you heat the pan, the water will begin to spatter at 100°C, which indicates that it is the right time to carefully add the piccata to the pan and fry it to a golden brown on both sides. If you cannot place the entire piccata at once into the pan, heat the oven to 160°C and keep the lightly fried piccata warm.

The right temperature is important: if the pan is too cool, the egg mixture sticks to the pan; if it is too hot, the egg mixture burns.

Fennel Potato Oven Vegetables

Ingredients: 2 potatoes (250 g), 1 large fennel bulb (250 g), salt, pepper, 2 tomatoes (250 g), 1 tbsp olive oil (5 g), ½ lemon, zest and juice

- Peel potatoes and cut potatoes and fennel into 1-cm cubes; mix with spices, lemon zest and juice, and olive oil; put in the oven for 20 minutes at 175°C.
- Cut tomatoes into 1-cm cubes and chop the fennel greens; fold fennel greens and tomatoes in with the potato–fennel mix and bake for another 10 minutes.

Pan-fried Vegetable Quinoa

Ingredients: 1 small onion (50 g), 1 medium-size zucchini (courgette) (200 g), 3 medium-size tomatoes (300 g), salt, pepper, 100 g quinoa, cooked, 2 tbsp basil, chopped, lemon zest, 1 tbsp olive oil (10 g), 1 tbsp parmesan (10 g)

- Dice onion and lightly sauté on medium heat without fat.
- Cut zucchini and tomatoes into 1-cm cubes, add to the onion and sauté for another 2 minutes.
- Add the cooked quinoa, the basil, and the lemon zest; sauté for an additional 5 minutes.
- At the end, add the olive oil, arrange on a plate and sprinkle with parmesan.

Pan-fried Carrot and Leek Millet

Ingredients: 3 carrots (450 g), 1 leek (100 g), 1 garlic clove, 2 thyme twigs, 1 cup of millet (125 g), 400 mL water, salt, pepper, 10 g olive oil, 2 tbsp basil, chopped

- Cut vegetables into small pieces and lightly sauté with the crushed garlic clove; add thyme and millet; continue to sauté for 2 minutes and deglaze with water.
- Continue to simmer for 10 minutes.
- Turn off heat and let it soak for another 5 minutes.
- Add salt and pepper to taste, add olive oil, and finish off with chopped basil.

Pan-fried Vegetable Millet

Ingredients: 1 small onion (50 g), 1 medium-size zucchini (courgette) (200 g), 3 medium-size tomatoes (300 g), salt, pepper, 100 g millet, cooked, 2 tbsp basil, chopped, lemon zest, 1 tbsp olive oil (10 g), 1 tbsp parmesan (10 g)

- Dice onion and lightly sauté on medium heat without fat.
- Cut zucchinis and tomatoes into 1-cm cubes, add to the onion and sauté for another 2 minutes.
- Add the cooked millet, the basil, and the lemon zest; sauté for additional 5 minutes.
- To finish, add the olive oil, arrange on a plate and sprinkle with parmesan.

▶ You need the same vegetable ingredients for the pan-fried vegetable quinoa as you do for the pan-fried vegetable millet.

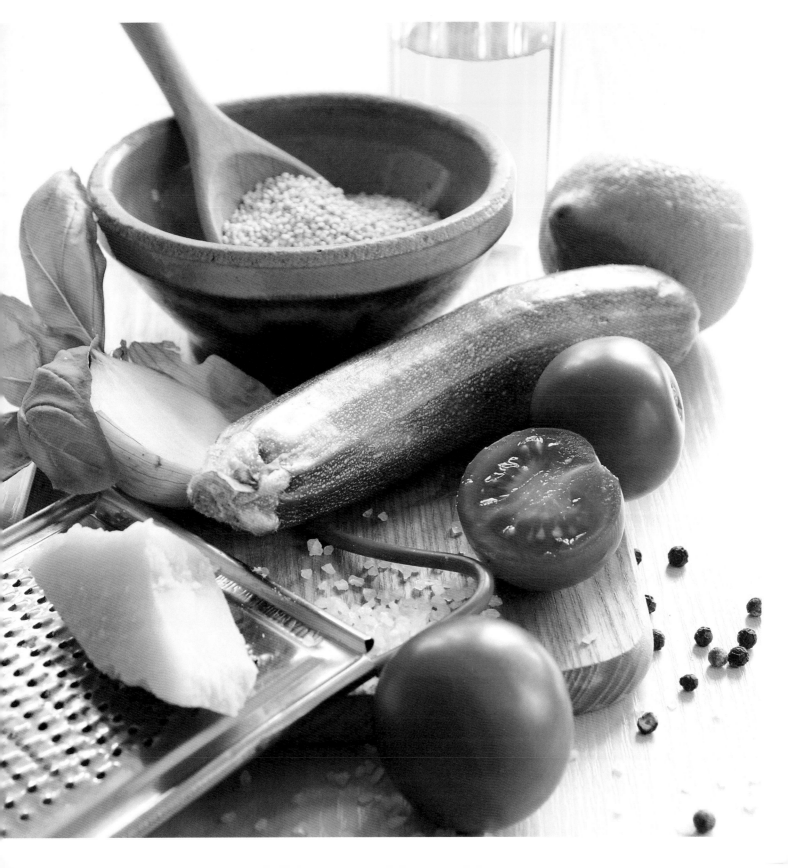

Zucchini Tomato Curry

Ingredients: 1 onion, 1 tsp olive oil, 1 zucchini (courgette), 2 tomatoes, vegetable broth or water, lemon zest, 1 tbsp mint, chopped, salt, pepper, 1 tsp curry powder

- Sauté finely diced onion in hot olive oil until translucent.
- Cut zucchini lengthwise, slice, and add to the onion with curry powder; sauté for 3 minutes; deglaze with some vegetable broth or water; season, cover, and continue sautéing until almost done.
- Cut tomatoes into eight pieces, add to the zucchini, and sauté for another 4 minutes. Sprinkle with chopped mint and lemon zest.

Polenta

Ingredients: 200 mL vegetable broth or water, salt, pepper, ¼ tsp curcuma (turmeric), 50 g polenta (cornmeal), 1 tbsp parmesan, grated (10 g), 1 tbsp tarragon

- Bring liquids to a boil in a pot and add spices. Pour polenta into the boiling liquid and stir well.
- Simmer on medium heat for 5 minutes.
- Add the grated parmesan and herbs and mix them in with the polenta, taste and possibly season again.
- Take a spoon and form small dumplings from the polenta. Serve, for example, with a vegetable dish.

Tip

Polenta is a nice side dish for the zucchini tomato curry.

Kohlrabi Saltimbocca

Ingredients: 2 kohlrabi (250 g), 2 tomatoes (200 g), salt, pepper, 60 g mozzarella, 10 sage leaves

- Peel the kohlrabi, slice, and steam until they are soft.
- Cut tomatoes into the same number of slices.
- Layer a heat-resistant casserole dish alternating with kohlrabi slices, sage leaves, and tomato slices; season with salt and pepper; cover with the mozzarella, which has been cut into small pieces.
- Bake in the oven at 175°C for 15 minutes.

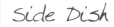

Side Dish

Rice, quinoa, or polenta go well with this dish.

Squash Risotto

Ingredients: 1 small onion, 100 g whole grain rice, ¼ tsp curry powder, 1 stalk of lemongrass, 400 mL water, 150 g squash (orange-colored Hokkaido), 200 mL milk (1.5% fat), salt, pepper, 10 g parmesan, finely grated

- Finely dice onion and gently roast in a pot; add rice, curry powder, and lemongrass, briefly sauté, add water.
- Cut squash into 1-cm cubes.
- Continue to cook rice for 20 minutes and then add squash and milk.
- Continue to simmer for an additional 10 minutes, check for desired consistency. When everything is soft, add salt and pepper to taste, and sprinkle with parmesan.

▶ This is what the kohlrabi saltimbocca looks like before placing it in the oven.

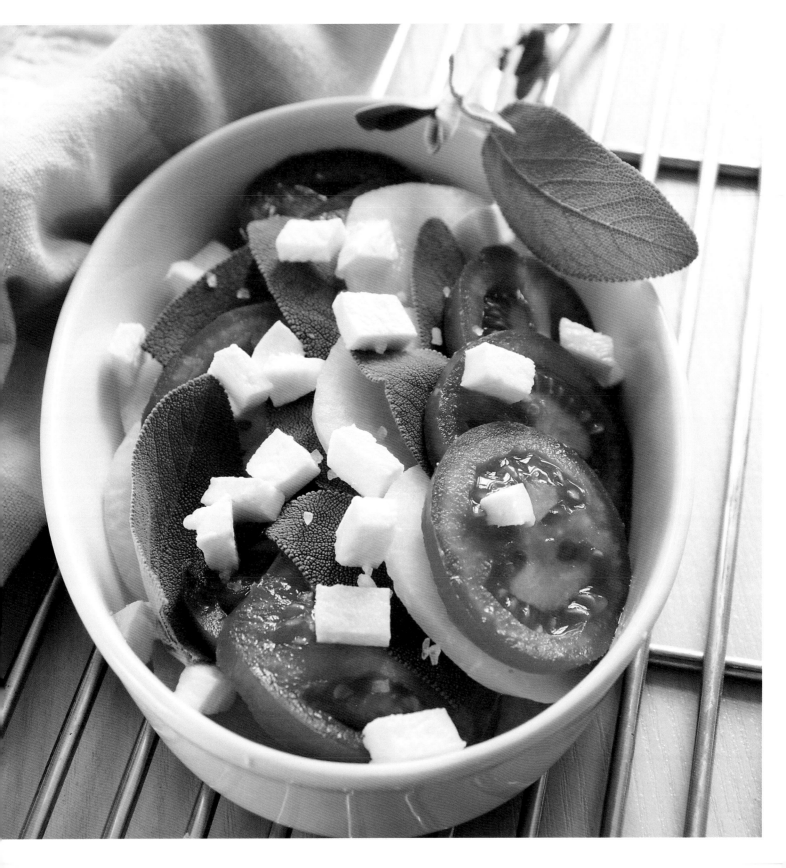

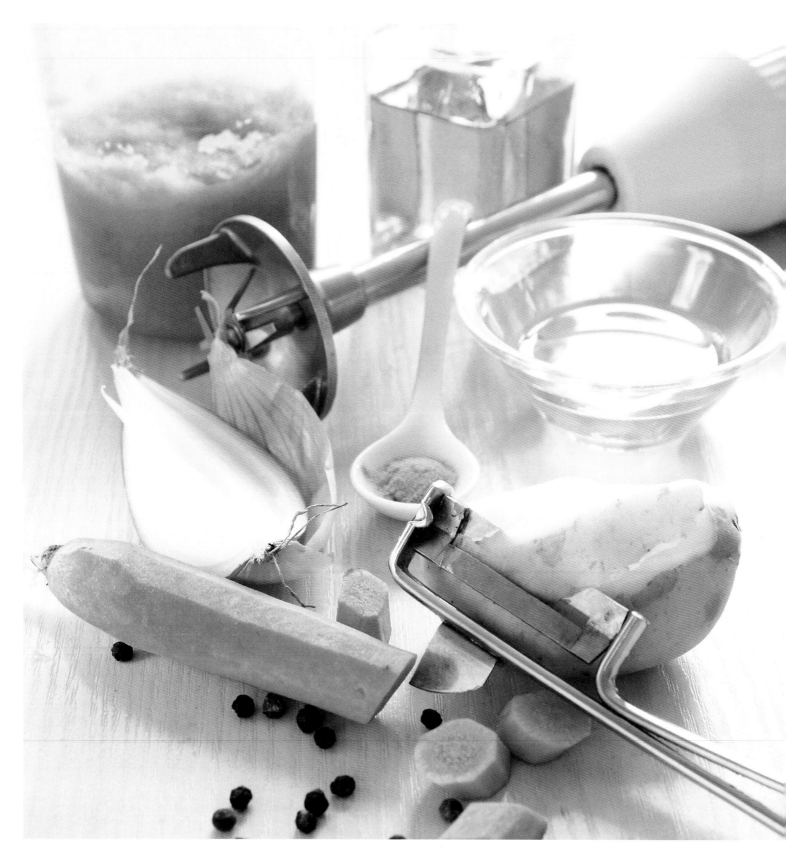

Sauces

The preparation of soups and sauces is identical. Today's pumpkin soup may be tomorrow's pumpkin sauce. Here is the difference: a soup is a dish by itself and should not be overly seasoned. A sauce, on the other hand, must sometimes provide the flavor for the entire dish—think about the great number of pasta dishes. When you use the following recipes to prepare sauces, feel free to make generous amounts as they are not thickeners. The basic sauce below is a true quick-change artist. Whether you combine it with herbs, mustard, saffron, horseradish, or cheese, this sauce always complements your dish.

Carrot Sauce

Ingredients: 1 tsp olive oil (5 g), ½ onion, 1 carrot (120 g), 1 small potato, peeled (50 g), 400 mL vegetable broth or water, 1 tbsp almond oil (10 g), some raspberry vinegar, salt, pepper, ¼ tsp curcuma (turmeric)

- Cut vegetables into walnut-size pieces, sauté with the curcuma in olive oil, deglaze with the liquid, season, and continue to cook until vegetables are soft.
- Purée in a blender until mix turns into a creamy, smooth sauce.
- Taste, add almond oil and raspberry vinegar and mix in.
- If the sauce is too thick, adjust the consistency with vegetable broth.

◄ The cooked ingredients for the carrot sauce are puréed in a blender to make a smooth sauce.

Basic Sauce

Ingredients: 1 tbsp olive oil (10 g), 60 g leek (only the white part), 50 g fennel, 40 g celery root, peeled, 40 g parsley root, peeled (or other white vegetable), 2 medium-size potatoes (220 g), 1 L water or light vegetable broth, salt, pepper, 1 bay leaf

- Chop the cleaned and rinsed vegetables into walnut-size cubes and lightly sauté in olive oil without browning.
- Add the liquid and bay leaf and cook until soft.
- Add salt and pepper to taste, add vegetable seasoning if necessary. Purée in a blender until the consistency is smooth and creamy.

This sauce can be used as a base and can be refined with flavoring ingredients, dairy products, or oils.

Classic Vinaigrette

Ingredients: 1 tsp mustard, salt, pepper, 50 mL vinegar (e.g., red wine vinegar), 1 garlic clove, crushed, 150 mL water, 80 mL cold-pressed oil (e.g., olive oil), 1 tbsp freshly chopped herbs

- Blend mustard, salt, and pepper with some vinegar until smooth and add garlic clove; now add the remaining vinegar, water, and oil and whisk.
- Finally, add freshly chopped herbs.

Tip

The choice of vegetable oil and vinegar determines the flavor of the vinaigrette.

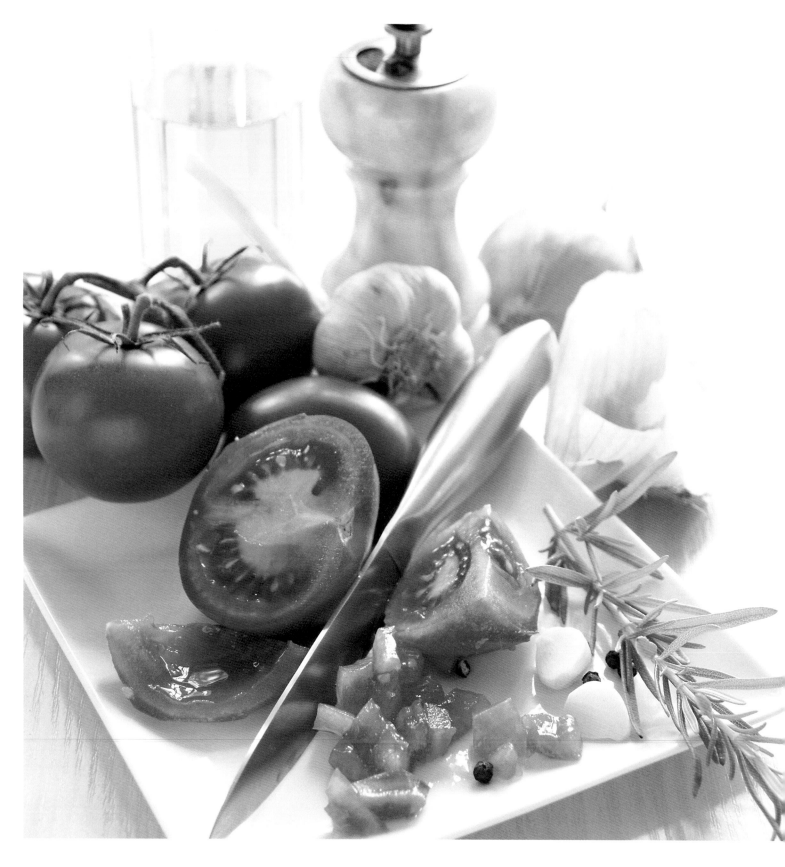

Tomato Vinaigrette

Ingredients: 5 ripe tomatoes, 20 mL balsamic vinegar, 1 small garlic clove, 100 mL vegetable broth, 50 mL olive oil, 10 basil leaves, salt, pepper

- Purée all ingredients, except the basil, in a blender until creamy. To finish, add the finely chopped basil.

Carrot Vinaigrette

Ingredients: 100 mL carrot juice, 50 mL nut oil, ¼ avocado (50 g), 20 mL apple cider vinegar, salt, pepper, 1 tbsp freshly chopped herbs (e.g., rucola [rocket], parsley, dill)

- Purée all ingredients, except the herbs, in a blender until the mix turns into an orange-colored, creamy sauce. To finish, add the finely chopped herbs.

Beetroot Sauce

Ingredients: 1 beetroot (120 g), 1 small potato, peeled (50 g), 20 g leek, 1 tsp olive oil (5 g), 400 mL vegetable broth, 1 bay leaf, 1 tbsp walnut oil (10 g), 1 tsp apple cider vinegar, 1 tsp horseradish, freshly shredded, salt, pepper

- Cut beetroot and potato into walnut-size cubes, finely slice leek, and lightly sauté everything in olive oil.
- Add the vegetable broth and bay leaf and cook on low heat until soft.
- Remove the bay leaf when everything is soft, purée in a blender. While purée-ing, add apple cider vinegar, horseradish, oil, and spices. Season to taste.
- If the sauce is too thick, adjust the consistency with vegetable broth.

Tomato Coulis

Ingredients: 500 g tomatoes, red and ripe, 2 small onions, 3 tbsp olive oil, 2 garlic cloves, crushed, salt, pepper, 1 twig of rosemary

- Peel tomatoes and remove seeds, chop into 1-cm cubes.
- Dice onions and lightly sauté in olive oil without browning them.
- Add garlic, cubed tomatoes, salt and pepper. Simmer for a few minutes. Add the rosemary twig, cover and allow to steep for at least 1 hour.

This recipe is very simple, but all ingredients, especially the tomatoes, must be high quality.

◄ Tomato coulis: the preparation is simple, but this dish needs to sit for 1 hour before serving.

Creative Salads

Salads should be the first course of a menu. Aside from fruit, which should be eaten as an in-between snack or for desert, salad provides us with fresh, nonheated food and is therefore important in regard to our vitamin supply.

Broccoli Pear Cashew Salad

Ingredients: 1 tbsp nut oil (10 g), 1 tbsp raspberry vinegar (10 g), juice of ½ orange, salt, pepper, 30 g cashew nuts, roasted and finely chopped or grated, 50 g yoghurt (1.5% fat), 1 broccoli (350 g), 1 pear (150 g)

- Blend the first five ingredients for the marinade. Add cashew nuts and stir in the yoghurt.
- Peel the stalk of the broccoli and mince broccoli with a knife or a grater. Grate the pear and combine everything with the marinade.

Cucumber Apple Salad

Ingredients: 1 tbsp walnut oil (10 g), 1 tbsp raspberry vinegar (10 g), salt, pepper, 1 cucumber (350 g), 1 apple (150 g), 1 tbsp mint

- Prepare the marinade by combining the oil, vinegar, and spices.
- Chop the cucumber and apple into 0.5-cm cubes, add to the marinade, mix in the mint and allow to infuse for ca. 10 minutes.

Leek in Vinaigrette Sauce

Ingredients: 400 g leek (use the white part only), 1 tsp mustard, salt, pepper, 20 mL white wine vinegar, 1 garlic clove, crushed, 50 mL water, 30 mL olive oil, 3 tbsp freshly chopped herbs

- This recipe serves four people.
- Cut leek lengthwise, rinse thoroughly, and cut into pieces of 10 cm. Steam leek until soft.
- For the vinaigrette, blend mustard, salt, and pepper with some vinegar until smooth; add garlic clove; whisk in remaining vinegar water, and oil.
- To finish, add freshly chopped herbs.
- The cooking time for the leek should allow the leek fibers to become tender. Drain the leek pieces well, pour the vinaigrette over the leek, and allow to infuse for ca. 30 minutes.

▶ Broccoli pear cashew salad.

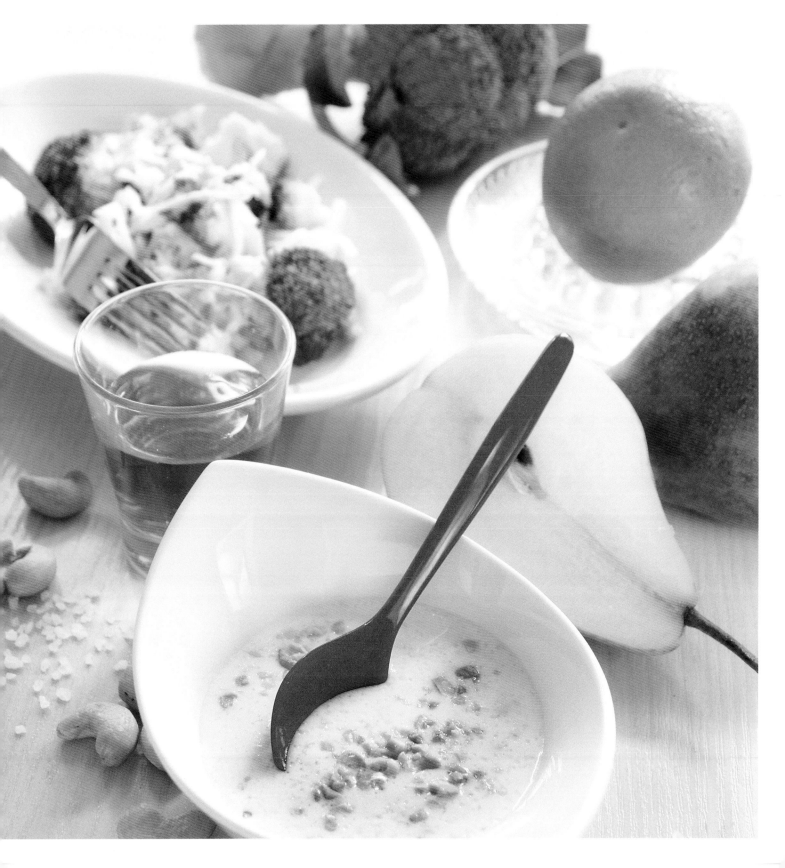

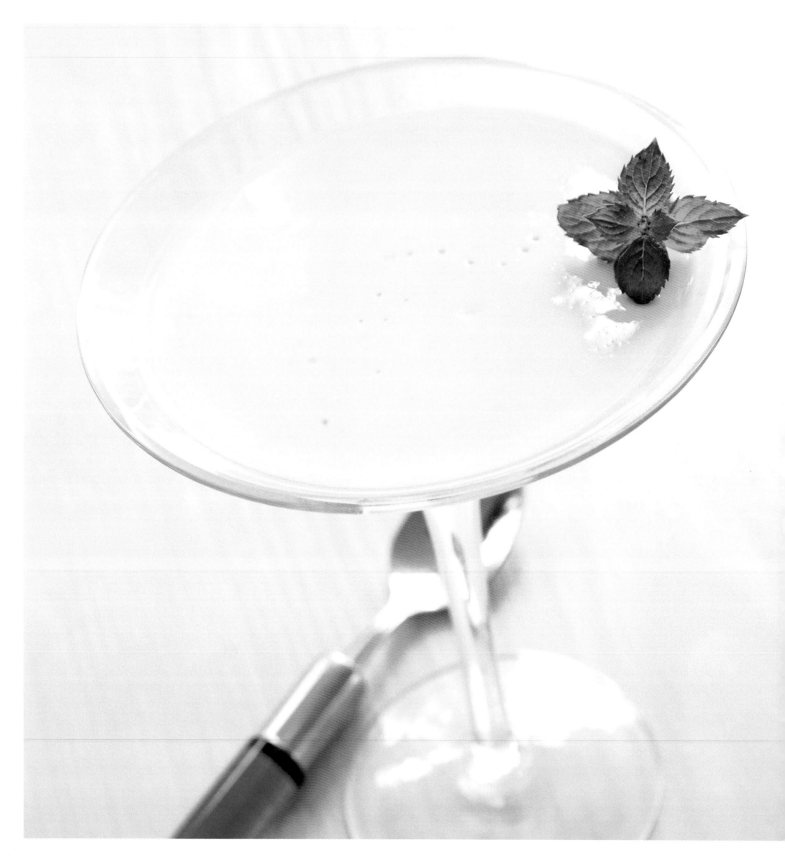

Sweet Treats

A tasty dessert is the enjoyable sweet conclusion, the highlight that tops off the menu. Ideally, the dessert should contain a large portion of fruit and be made of low-fat dairy products. Preferably, avoid cream and large amounts of sugar.

Fruit Crumble

Ingredients: 250 g wheat, ground, 200 g brown sugar, 100 g almonds, grated, 100 mL almond oil, 2 apples, cut into quarters and sliced, cinnamon, vanilla

- Recipe for one baking dish (serves four people).
- Mix wheat, brown sugar, and grated almonds; add almond oil and crumble with your hands (i.e., let the mix trickle through your fingers, applying light pressure, until you have crumble).
- Flavor the cut fruit with cinnamon and vanilla, place in lightly greased baking dish, sprinkle the crumble over the fruit, and bake in the oven at 160°C for ca. 30 minutes.
- Best served with vanilla sauce.

Tip

Pineapples, bananas, or pears are great replacements for the apples.

Mango Cream

Ingredients: 250 mL mango juice, 1 tbsp honey, $^1/_3$ tsp agar-agar, 150 g low-fat quark (room temperature), vanilla or 1 star anise, ginger, clover, cinnamon

- Recipe serves four people.
- Bring mango juice, spices, and agar-agar to a boil; allow to cool to 35°C.
- Bring the low-fat quark to room temperature and whisk with a hand-held mixer. Mix everything together, pour into a dish and store in a cool place.

Vanilla Cream

Ingredients: 250 mL milk, 1 tbsp brown sugar, 20 g pumpkin, finely shredded, ½ tsp natural vanilla, 25 g whole-grain rice, ground

- Recipe serves two people.
- While heating the milk, stir in sugar, shredded pumpkin, vanilla, and ground rice; bring to a boil while stirring, and continue to boil for 2 minutes.
- Taste and pour into small dishes.

Tip

Vanilla cream can be served with raspberry or strawberry sauce, and fresh fruit.

◀ Vanilla cream

Cocktails

You can create interesting cocktails from fruit juices, teas, and herbs. They can have a refreshing, fruity, or exotic flavor and be pleasing to the eye. It goes without saying that they do not need alcohol or sugar.

Mallow Infusion

Ingredients: 1 L water, 1 tbsp mallow tea, 5 mint leaves, ½ orange, ½ lemon (natural fruits, as the zest is used as well)

- Pour water and all other ingredients into a sealable container and allow to infuse for 2 days in a cool place; after 2 days simply strain. This infusion may be kept refrigerated for several days.
- You may dilute it with up to 2 parts mineral water, as desired.

If you do not have the required time, you may use a quarter of the water and let everything simmer on low heat for 20 minutes. Take cold water and fill up to 1 L.

Colorful Cocktail

Ingredients: 80 mL apple-mango juice (from a health food store), 40 mL mallow infusion, 140 mL mineral water

- This amount fills two champagne glasses.
- Pour equal parts of the apple-mango juice into the two champagne glasses.
- Mix the mallow infusion with the mineral water.
- Hold a curved spoon directly above the apple-mango juice in the glass and carefully pour the mallow-water mixture on top of it. The goal is to create a bi-colored cocktail.

Avocado Cocktail

Ingredients: ½ avocado, 5 lemon basil leaves, 100 mL pineapple juice, 200 mL orange juice, 600 mL water

- Place all ingredients into a blender and mix well. Strain and serve cold.

Instead of lemon basil you may use basil and lemon balm.

Apple-Mango Drink

Ingredients: 1 apple, ½ mango, 1 tsp cinnamon, 2 cloves, 1 L water

- Cut apple with its peel into small cubes or shred it coarsely. Cut the mango into small cubes as well; add cinnamon and cloves, mix, and add the water. Simmer for 15 minutes and then allow to steep for 10 minutes.

This drink may be served cold or hot. You may sweeten with some honey, as desired.

▶ Cool, tea-based cocktails are refreshing and low in calories.

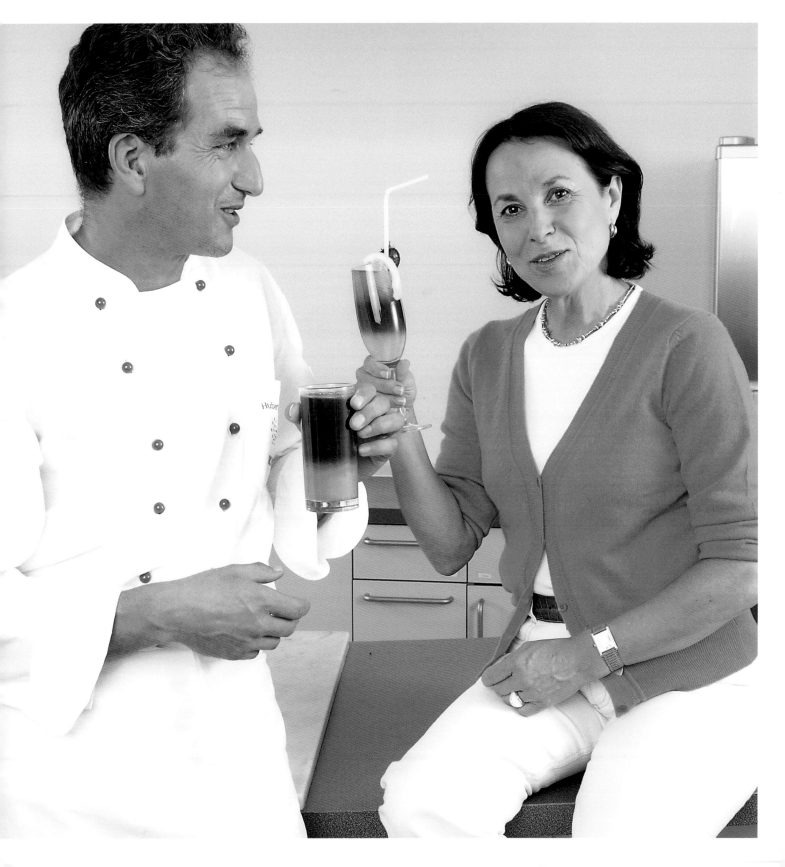